Exercising
Through Your
Pregnancy

James F. Clapp III, M.D.

Addicus Books
Omaha, Nebraska

An Addicus Nonfiction Book

ISBN# 1-886039-59-3-1
Cover design by Peri Paloni

This book is not intended to serve as a substitute for a physician. Nor does the author intend to give medical advice contrary to that of an attending physician's.

Library of Congress Cataloging-in-Publication Data

Clapp, James F., 1936-
  Exercising through your pregnancy / James F. Clapp III.
    p. cm.
  Includes bibliographical references and index.
  ISBN 1-886039-59-3
  1. Exercise for pregnant women. I. Title.
RG558.7 .C58 2002
618.2'4—dc21

                                        2001007237

Addicus Books, Inc.
P.O. Box 45327
Omaha, Nebraska 68145
Web site: http://www.AddicusBooks.com

Printed in the United States of America
10 9 8 7 6 5 4 3 2 1

To my mother and father for teaching me to be inquisitive and to my wife, Nancy, and my children, James, Andrew, and Elizabeth, for indulging me and supporting the time commitment necessary to conduct the research for this book.

Contents

Preface

I am blessed by a curiosity that leads me to take an offbeat approach to scientific inquiry. Rather than studying an isolated variable in a controlled environment, I like to study whole individuals in their environments and the complex interactions that occur in these environments and observe what happens. I used this approach when I began studying exercise during pregnancy, and it produced different answers than either I or others had anticipated. As these answers have broad health-related implications for pregnant women and their offspring, it seems important to pass them on to those most affected: women anticipating or experiencing pregnancy and their health care and fitness providers.

This book details my firsthand experiences studying over 250 women who exercised regularly before, during, and after pregnancy and another group of more than 50 women who began one of several structured exercise programs during pregnancy. These studies were broad, in-depth investigations that focused on the multiple effects of regular exercise before, during, and immediately after pregnancy that create concern for the women themselves and for those who supervise their athletic endeavors and their medical care. The studies detail what these healthy women did before, during, and after pregnancy and what effect it had on them, their pregnancies, and their offspring—as newborns and throughout their first five years of life. As such, the studies give a comprehensive picture of what happens to exercise performance and the reproductive process when a woman continues, starts, or stops a regular exercise regimen during the months when she is trying to get pregnant, as well as during the various stages of pregnancy and lactation.

The results of these studies cast serious doubt on many old myths and concerns about exercising during pregnancy and shed new insight on the interaction among exercise, health, fitness, and the course and outcome of pregnancy. For example, many active women have been warned by others that regular exercise probably interferes with a woman's ability to get pregnant and can cause an early miscarriage or premature labor. Likewise, most health care professionals believe that vigorous weight-bearing exercise during late pregnancy and in the first few weeks after the birth probably damages ligaments and other connective tissues causing long-term problems with joint stability, abdominal muscle tone, bladder control, and sexual function. However, the results to date negate most concerns in these and many other areas.

Exercising Through Your Pregnancy not only provides the physically active, healthy woman with the information she needs to understand the effects of regular exercise on the reproductive process, so she can appropriately plan her physical activity during conception, pregnancy, and lactation, but also speaks to health care and fitness professionals—physical trainers, coaches, fitness instructors, nurses, midwives, doctors, health club personnel, physical therapists, nutritionists, and so on—who interact with physically active women. This book guides these professionals to develop a rational, objective, and individualized approach to both exercise prescription, exercise monitoring, and pregnancy care for different groups of physically active women. Finally, the book discusses in detail the past and current controversies that surround continuing strenuous exercise during the process of conceiving, carrying, birthing, and nursing a baby, which should provide valuable reading for family members including fathers-to-be or grandparents-to-be who are anxious about the effects of exercise during pregnancy on the mother and baby.

I've divided the book into three parts to clearly separate the myths, concerns, and other essential background information from new factual information and to provide a section focusing on issues related to exercise prescription. Part I provides information about the concerns surrounding exercise and reproduction and the interesting interactions among physical activity and ovulation, pregnancy, lactation, and recovery from the birthing process. Part II details the effects of exercise on fertility, miscarriage, congenital defects, other abnormalities of fetal growth, labor, the mother-to-be, her recovery, lactation, and the growth and development of her offspring through early childhood. Part III draws from the information provided in parts I and II to formulate principles I recommend health care or fitness professionals and the pregnant woman use to develop a practical approach to designing a holistic, individualized exercise program that includes monitoring for each phase of the reproductive process.

This book's three parts provide women and health fitness professionals with a working knowledge and healthy perspective about the interactions among various levels and patterns of physical activity and the various phases of the reproductive process. I focus on three groups of exercising women: the beginner, the recreational athlete (someone who exercises at a moderate intensity for 20 to 60 minutes, 3 to 7 times per week), and the competitive athlete (someone who regularly works out at varying levels of intensity, 8 to 14 times per week). I also provide detailed information about the physically active woman who does not engage in a strenuous, sustained, exercise routine, but who occasionally walks, gardens, or plays tennis, racquetball, or golf. The research protocols also examine what happens when a woman stops or cuts way back on her exercise program in mid- or late pregnancy.

Exercising Through Your Pregnancy can help the active woman and her health or fitness professional merge basic principles with the practical tools needed to develop an appropriate program of exercise and monitoring. By appropriate, I mean one that safely fulfills an individual's specific needs during the different phases of the reproductive process (the preconceptional period; early, mid-, and late pregnancy; the first six weeks after the birth; and the remainder of lactation). Parts I and II present background to enable a woman and her fitness and health care providers to evaluate new information about exercise and reproduction as it appears and to incorporate this new research into their approach to exercise during the reproductive process. The book also provides readers with information to make the interactions between physically active women and their health care providers easier and more positive. Finally, I hope the knowledge and understanding of the topic increases confidence and diminishes apprehension and guilt about maintaining or incorporating a regular exercise regimen into daily life during the reproductive process.

Although I did not specifically write this book for physicians or researchers, it does include an extensive bibliography for the interested reader. I, however, purposely do not address the role of exercise in chronic disease states during pregnancy in detail because, right now, little is known. Although the chapters about exercise prescription (part III) detail contraindications to exercise for *normal healthy* women in all three groups (beginner, recreational, and competitive athletes), they do not provide guidelines for women with underlying chronic disease, nor do they discuss what to do during acute illness. Both situations require detailed medical evaluation that is not usually required, and women who experience either should consult their personal physicians or obstetricians before beginning or continuing a regular exercise program.

Acknowledgments

None of this would have been possible without the interest and dedication of the women who participated in the exercise in pregnancy study I conducted over the last 10 years. I give a heartfelt thanks to them and their spouses who all gave so freely of themselves, their time, their privacy, and their offspring.

A big thank you to Rob Sleamaker, Carol Van Dyke, and Pat Bannerman for all their help, interest, and encouragement along the way, and to all the others who contributed so much to the success of the laboratory studies dealing with exercise in pregnancy:

Early Days in Vermont
Rob Sleamaker, MS
Rod Larrow, BA
Brian Seaward, PhD
Lorraine Betz, MS
John Hiser, MS
Cissy Capeless, MD
Chrissa Philbin, RD

Recent Years in Ohio
Kathy Little, PhD
Pat Gott, RD
Karen Rizk, MS, RN
Sarah Appleby-Wineberg, MS
Susan Ridzon, MS, RD
Beth Lopez, RN
Jodi Tomaselli, MS

A special word of thanks to Dr. Leon Mann who served as my departmental chairman at both places. His support was invaluable. Without it I never would have had the necessary time, space, people, and equipment to explore in detail the issue of exercise in pregnancy.

Many thanks also to the numerous physicians, midwives, and nurses throughout Vermont, New Hampshire, and Ohio who were so helpful to us as they rendered care to these women.

Finally, much of the work would not have been possible without the financial support of the National Institutes of Health, the National Foundation March of Dimes, the Harry W. Chandler and Grace F. Clapp Memorial Research Funds, the Alexander von Humboldt Foundation, and funds from MetroHealth Medical Center.

PART I

Why Exercise During Pregnancy?

When researching in a field of study, it's always wise to begin at the beginning so you can trace the evolution of thought about it and understand what is and what is not known, what appears to be important, and why. This part of the book is designed to do precisely that for active women and their health and fitness professionals. It provides a historical overview of research dealing with exercise during pregnancy and prepares the reader for parts II and III by explaining essential biological and physiological information of exercise during pregnancy. Chapter 1 traces the origins and development of the two opposite opinions about exercise during pregnancy:

1. It is probably very bad for the mother and baby.
2. It is probably very good for the mother and baby.

The first opinion is often held by doctors as well as grandmothers-to-be, leading them to take a more restrictive approach to prescribing or condoning exercise for pregnant women. The second opinion has often been held by already active women, leading them to take a more liberal approach to exercising during their pregnancies. The obvious conflict between these two opinions led me to begin serious studies concerning the effects of exercise on pregnancy. Chapter 2 details the basics of the changes that occur in various physiological systems in a woman's body during pregnancy and during exercise and then discusses why the changes produced by exercise are actually helpful to the pregnancy, and vice versa. This is a key chapter because its conclusions coupled with the study results presented in part II are the basis for the approach to exercise prescription discussed in part III.

CHAPTER 1

Clarifying the Debate Over Exercise and Pregnancy

B ack in the early 1970s, the University of Vermont Information Service asked me to contact a rural doctor who had called inquiring about the effects of mountain climbing on a woman and her fetus during early pregnancy. The note said he wanted to know if the decreased oxygen in the rarefied air might induce malformations in the fetus. Would the intense effort climbing required reduce blood flow to the womb and cause a miscarriage? Was localized pressure from the climbing harness likely to cause a problem?

I had no ready answers to these questions, so I went directly to the library and soon found out there weren't any. Nor were there answers to obvious questions about the safety of the many forms of recreational exercise during pregnancy. There were only a few case studies of women who exercised during pregnancy without incident, similar anecdotal reports of pregnancy outcome in some Olympic and national class athletes, and evidence that size at birth was slightly reduced in the offspring of women who lived at altitudes above 1,600 meters. Nonetheless, most books dealing with pregnancy and childbirth expressed the view that pregnancy was a time for moderation, and a woman should not introduce new activity or attempt anything physically challenging during pregnancy.

Early Studies

I was amazed! Why didn't we know much more about the effects of strenuous physical activity on the unborn baby and mother? Clearly we needed some answers. My next stop was the physiology laboratory where, in 1976, we began experiments to determine if strenuous maternal exercise was potentially harmful to the unborn baby. Over the next few months, we exercised a group of near-term pregnant sheep on a treadmill and observed the responses of the mother and unborn lamb to strenuous exercise.

I never will forget the start of the first experiment. We began our measurements with a ewe standing quietly in a plywood pen on the treadmill. Then she began walking slowly at one mile per hour up a three-percent grade, but absolutely nothing happened to her heart rate, blood pressure, respiration, or the rate of blood flow to the placenta and fetus. I doubled the speed and she simply looked calmly at me over the top of the pen, so up went the speed and the grade. Still nothing happened. All I could hear was the sound of the treadmill running and the sound of the ewe chewing her cud. She wasn't even breathing hard; something had to be wrong. I stood up and looked over the edge of the plywood at the treadmill belt. It was moving quite rapidly but the ewe wasn't. She was straddling the belt with one point of each of her cloven hoofs balanced on the narrow, quarter-inch rim of the treadmill deck!

Once we rebuilt the pen so the ewes couldn't cheat, we found that strenuous exercise in these placid animals rapidly increased maternal body temperature to high levels and decreased the rate of blood flow to the placenta and fetus by more than 50 percent (Clapp 1980). Although both responses were dramatic and potentially harmful, the unborn lambs handled them well for an hour of continuous exercise, indicating that the lamb and its placenta were able to compensate even under demanding circumstances. Although sheep are clearly not people, these findings were both reassuring and consistent with the findings meager amounts of research had shown in humans, so I shifted my attention to other things.

Early animal experiments demonstrated that the fetus tolerated the thermal and circulatory stresses of exercise well in late pregnancy.

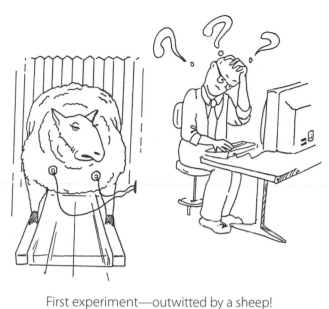

First experiment—outwitted by a sheep!

Several years later, other investigators, who were motivated by similar concerns, performed more detailed experiments in pregnant ewes (Lotgering, Gilbert, and Longo 1983a, 1983b). They exercised the ewes for different periods of time at various workloads and measured several additional functions, including the exercise-induced decrease in maternal blood volume, which usually accentuates the decrease in blood flow to the placenta and fetus, and fetal temperature. Again, although the changes observed in temperature, blood volume, and blood flow were dramatic and potentially harmful, the lambs showed no evidence of distress, even when the ewes exercised near their maximal capacities for protracted periods. Other laboratories examined several additional cardiovascular and hormonal responses to acute exercise in the same animal model with similar findings. Later in the decade, two reviews were published that synthesized the information obtained in these and other experiments (Clapp 1987; Lotgering, Gilbert, and Longo 1985). They reached three conclusions.

1. Acute exercise during pregnancy had dramatic effects on maternal physiology without producing evidence of a detrimental effect on the animal fetus late in pregnancy.

2. Almost nothing was known about the fetal effects of maternal exercise in the human, and they would probably be different because of species differences in posture (quadruped versus biped), thermoregulation

(respiratory heat loss versus sweating), placental type and function, and cardiovascular responses.

3. Despite the reassuring findings in large animals, studies in humans would be required before the multiple questions about the safety of exercise during pregnancy for women and fetuses could be answered.

Attitudes About Exercising During Pregnancy

Over this time (the late 1970s and early 1980s), women's interest in regular physical activity grew rapidly, and, as a result, recreational exercise became an integral part of life for an increasing number of women. Interest in various forms of recreational exercise spread and, in my area of the country, it reached explosive proportions in the early 1980s. The number of inquiries and concerns about exercising throughout pregnancy grew steadily, and the pressure for answers, or at least sensible guidance, grew rapidly. Doctors and other health care providers wanted something concrete to tell their patients, and active women wanted definite answers. Inevitably, in response to these pressures for a definite opinion, two divergent schools of thought evolved. Unfortunately, both were based primarily on theory, speculation, or anecdotal experience.

Most individuals over the age of 40 and most health care providers shared the more conservative, or no-risk, view. Their point of view was expressed in the contraindications to and guidelines for exercise in pregnancy published in 1985 by the American College of Obstetricians and Gynecologists (ACOG) and in the first text dealing specifically with exercise in pregnancy (Artal and Wiswell 1986). Both detailed the theoretical risks to mother and fetus and recommended that active women stringently limit the type, duration, and intensity of their exercise during pregnancy to minimize maternal and fetal risk. As the national body responsible for female reproductive care sanctioned this approach, it immediately became the standard of care, providing doctors with a concrete approach. These guidelines have recently been revised and liberalized to some degree (American College of Obstetricians and Gynecologists 1994). In philosophy and practical application, however, it appears they are basically unchanged (Artal 1996; Artal and Buckenmeyer 1995). Chapter 8 includes a synopsis of these traditional, conservative guidelines as well as a list of their warning signs and contraindications to exercise.

The opposite, more liberal view was espoused by many physically active women who had maintained vigorous exercise regimens throughout pregnancy and experienced trouble-free pregnancies, followed by easy labors and quick recoveries. These women argued that historical perspective did not support the conservative avoidance approach and maintained that regular physical activity at levels well above those recommended did no harm, would reduce pregnancy complications, improve well-being, shorten labor, and speed recovery for most women with normal pregnancies.

Predictably, the evolution of these two opinions without new information forced most individuals interested in the area to assume one of the two polarized views, which did not resolve anything. Rather, it created a greater dilemma as well as a new set of subliminal fears for the physically active woman planning pregnancy. On the one hand, she wanted to believe that she could maintain her activity level without risk to the pregnancy. On the other, she was uncertain if it was really safe, and the concerns voiced by many well meaning individuals around her—mother, mother-in-law, friends, neighbors, even the butcher and grocery clerk—constantly reinforced this uncertainty. As yet, time and a great deal of new information has not really helped this problem of perception. It is hoped the information in this book will. The following list illustrates some of the currently voiced questions, uncertainties, and concerns that are answered later in this book.

- Does high-impact aerobics or swimming using flip turns cause the baby to get wrapped in its umbilical cord?
- Does the repetitive jarring of running and jumping cause the egg to tear loose from the wall of the womb in early pregnancy?
- Does exercise cause the bag of waters around the baby to burst ahead of schedule?
- Will exercise otherwise hurt the baby?
- Do strong pelvic muscles prolong the pushing phase of labor and make a forceps delivery necessary?
- Does strenuous exercise cause a mother's milk to taste sour and dry up?
- Will returning to exercise a week or two after the birth damage the abdominal wall or disturb the support of the bladder, vagina, and womb?

I should point out that life was not necessarily any easier on the clinical or practitioner side of the fence. In reality, doctors and midwives faced the same dilemma and had similar questions with no clear answers. However, they had the additional problem of potential lawsuits if they condoned an exercise regimen exceeding the ACOG sanctioned guidelines and a problem developed for either the mother or baby later in the pregnancy, whether the problem was truly related to the exercise regimen or not.

As you can imagine, this created a less than ideal doctor-patient relationship for the active woman and her health care provider. In 1984, a study done by one of our residents demonstrated how serious the rift was (Clapp and Dickstein 1984). All the women who registered for pregnancy care over a three-month interval were interviewed twice during pregnancy, and their charts were reviewed after delivery. Not one of the 96 pregnant women who exercised three or more times a week discussed it with any of the eight doctors who cared for them, and none of the doctors asked about exercise at any point during the pregnancy. Clearly, concern over the dilemma led both sides to adopt a "don't ask, don't tell" approach to the issue of exercise during pregnancy.

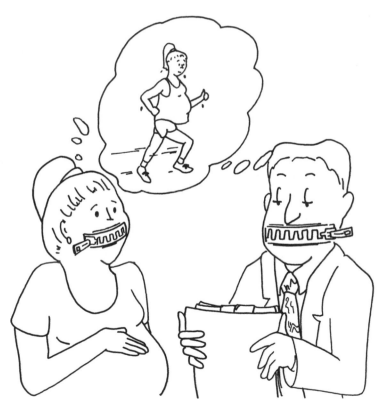

Don't ask, don't tell.

Origins of the Debate

I often ask myself, How could this state of affairs have come to be? A lot was known about the benefits of exercise. Historically, healthy women regularly performed hard physical work for prolonged periods while conceiving, carrying, delivering, and nursing their offspring without apparent harm, and the same was true for mammals in general. Tigresses continue to hunt, squirrels to forage and climb, and whales to swim and dive. So, if strenuous physical activity is a normal part of life, why all the fuss when women decide to exercise or train during pregnancy and lactation? The answer has both a societal and a biological bent.

Societal Origins

The fuss or avoidance response to women exercising during pregnancy represents the traditional, knee-jerk, societal response to an unknown risk. In this case, it reflects the underlying fear that exercise will harm the pregnancy or the woman. This may sound ridiculous, but an avoidance response to the unknown is deeply rooted in both medical and societal thought.

The traditional approach to an unknown risk is avoidance.

For all concerned, the logic goes this way. First, there is an anecdotal observation. For example, an infertility specialist notes at a meeting that many women she sees who have difficulty conceiving also exercise. Then she reaches a speculative conclusion and applies it generally (i.e., many women who exercise regularly will have trouble getting pregnant when they want to). The reality is that nobody knows if women who exercise regularly have more trouble getting pregnant than those who do not. Likewise, most people who lead a physically active lifestyle know of at least one woman runner, aerobicizer, swimmer, weight trainer, or the like who has had a miscarriage. Although nobody talks about it, everybody, including the woman, speculates that maybe the strenuous exercise caused the miscarriage.

The reality, however, is that miscarriage is a common occurrence (at least one in five pregnancies end that way), and nobody knows whether women who exercise miscarry more frequently or not. Nonetheless, as a conservative solution, many women and practitioners assume that a causal relationship exists and therefore restrict activity.

The answer to why the fuss is more complicated because it also reflects an avoidance approach to the issue of safety that has evolved within many groups for different reasons. For instance, not a day goes by without some lay or professional group publicizing another environmental or lifestyle factor that may threaten our well-being. They usually advise us what is best to do and not to do and what to eat and not eat to lessen our risk of this and that. Indeed, many ultimately wind up as law (package labeling, seat belts, helmets, infant car restraints, and so forth). Although their concern is genuine and the advice well meaning and often lifesaving, the subliminal message is "Be careful!" in all aspects of your life. Avoid as many potential threats as possible, and you will live a longer and healthier life. As a result, we live in a society where many drink bottled water, avoid all stimulants, use air purification systems, and avoid stress whenever possible. The same avoidance philosophy has become a central theme in the preventive aspects of medical and obstetrical care.

In addition, there is a generational gap in attitudes toward physical activity for women, especially during pregnancy and lactation. As a result, public health policies have slowed progress in the area. Although regular exercise is an asset to general health, and a public health goal is to have 90 percent or more of women of all ages regularly engage in sustained recreational exercise by the year 2000, most policy makers view women who are pregnant or lactating differently from those who are not. For example, when I presented carefully gathered preliminary data on the course and outcome of pregnancy in a group of women who had exercised regularly throughout pregnancy at a grant site visit, the members of the governmental site-visit team raised ethical issues about the research project. Despite information to the contrary, they felt that strenuous exercise during pregnancy was probably harmful, that I must have had a vested interest, and that, on ethical grounds, the research should not be allowed to continue. That was the mid-1980s, but I often hear similar opinions today.

The regulations governing physical activity in the workplace during pregnancy and the instructional guidelines given to prenatal educators are based on the same conservative principles. Presumably, this reflects the multiple legal concerns that a more liberal approach would generate in an area in which knowledge is limited.

Biological Origins

The first biological support for the fuss probably was the undeniable evidence that many things that mothers-to-be do or do not do can have short- and long-term effects on the pregnancy. This began in the 1950s with the diethylstilbestrol (D.E.S.) story. People were shocked to learn that hormonal treatment with D.E.S. for bleeding in early pregnancy produced a high incidence of reproductive tract malformations in the offspring, which increased the risk of reproductive difficulty and cancer later in their lives. Then in the 1960s, reports appeared from abroad that ingestion of a commonly prescribed sedative, thalidomide, was responsible for a variety of defects in heart and limb development. Then came smoking, alcohol ingestion, drug abuse, nutritive deficiencies, and so on. As a result, by the late 1970s and early 1980s, the perspective of both women and their health care providers began to shift from "pregnancy is a normal part of life" to "pregnancy is risky." Indeed, many women in westernized societies wondered if anything in their usual lifestyle would really be safe to do or ingest during pregnancy.

Concern about exercise during pregnancy grew when it became apparent that many things women did or did not do affected pregnancy outcome.

This view was strongly reinforced in the minds of women who regularly (three or more times each week) performed one or more types of sustained (20 minutes or more a session), strenuous (over 55 percent of their maximum intensity), weight-bearing exercise because a variety of findings in both experimental animals and men suggested that these forms of exercise might be harmful to the unborn baby. For example, during sustained bouts of strenuous exercise, researchers observed that blood flow to the internal organs of men fell by at least 50 percent, and body temperature often rose by more than 1.5 degrees centigrade (Grimby 1965; Rowell 1974; Saltin and Hermansen 1966; Snellen 1969). In addition, when blood flow to the womb was experimentally reduced in animal models throughout late pregnancy, it reduced the growth rate of the fetus. Moreover, extremely prolonged increases in body temperature in early pregnancy increased the incidence of congenital malformations. These findings raised two obvious questions: Would the transient decreases in blood flow to the womb during exercise slow the growth of the baby or restrict its oxygen supply? Would brief increases in the mother's temperature initiate fetal malformations?

More recently, yet another question was raised by the findings of several French and one American study. Their findings strongly suggested that high levels of physical stress in the workplace during pregnancy are associated with an increased rate of pregnancy complications, including premature birth (Clapp 1996c; Luke et al. 1995; Mamelle, Laumon, and Lazar 1984). Many reasoned "Why wouldn't the physical stress of exercise during pregnancy have the same effect?"

Likewise, information from automobile accidents indicated that either sudden deceleration or direct blows to the abdomen can cause direct injury to the unborn baby and its placenta. Why wouldn't the forces associated with sudden moves during exercise or an unanticipated fall do the same?

Finally, what about the mother herself? Shouldn't the well known, pregnancy-associated changes in body weight, posture, center of gravity, and relaxation of pelvic ligaments increase her risk of injury (Sherer and Schenker 1989)?

Theoretical Issues

This type of information and the questions it generated led to the development of what I call a *guilt by association* list of the theoretical problems that regular exercise during pregnancy might create in a variety of areas. Unfortunately, what now appears to be overconcern led well meaning individuals to put all the exercise-induced changes that anyone thought might possibly cause any problem for either the fetus or the mother on that list. That list soon became a part of common but, in most instances, unsubstantiated "knowledge" within the medical and sport science communities. Fortunately, the list had a catalytic effect as it clearly identified a large number of issues that piqued the interest of certain individuals. Once these individuals began to question the validity of items on this list, it stimulated research, which produced knowledge based on fact that resolved many issues of concern.

In the area of exercise and reproduction, the guilt by association list was a long one. Indeed, when the entire reproductive cycle was examined, clinical problems that exercise theoretically might cause or magnify were identified in each of its main phases (Clapp 1994a). For example, there were many areas in which regular exercise might interfere with conception. First, the increase in body temperature during exercise might increase the temperature of a man's testicles and kill developing sperm (especially if he wears Lycra tights). The same might be true for a woman's eggs. Second, the stress of training for serious competition clearly suppressed ovulation and menstruation for protracted periods in many national and international class female athletes. This might also be the case in women who exercised recreationally at much lower levels. Third, less severe disturbances in ovarian function and hormonal levels might alter the *receptivity* of the womb and interfere with the ability of a fertilized egg to implant normally in its wall.

There also were many concerns that exercise during early pregnancy would have harmful embryonic effects because, during sustained, strenuous exercise in the nonpregnant state, both body temperature and the levels of stress hormones rise and the rate of blood flow to the internal organs falls dramatically. During the first 12 weeks of pregnancy, these changes might initiate a variety of clinical problems such as miscarriage, abnormal implantation or ectopic pregnancy (in the tube, abdomen, or cervix), congenital malformations of the baby, and abnormalities in placental growth and development.

The list of apparent reasons not to exercise was even longer for women in late pregnancy. The clinical problems that might have a connection with exercise included back pain, loss of bladder control, abdominal hernia, premature labor, premature membrane rupture, infection, poor growth of the unborn baby, oxygen deprivation of the baby with brain damage, difficult labor, entanglement of the baby in its umbilical cord, distress in labor, and respiratory, thermoregulatory, and metabolic problems for the baby in the newborn period.

In the immediate period after birth, it was commonly thought that clinical problems that exercise might precipitate or aggravate were primarily maternal. They included heavy bleeding, anemia, fatigue, abdominal and vaginal hernias, poor healing, joint pain, traumatic arthritis, and ligamentous laxity with an increased risk of joint dislocation.

The final area in which there were concerns about exercise causing a clinical problem was lactation. Here, the issue was that exercise would decrease the quality and quantity of breast milk with subsequent effects on infant growth and development. For example, if the woman let herself get dehydrated, would the volume of milk decrease? Would it decrease the fatty acid content, alter the taste, and so forth?

The Stimulus for Research

By the mid-1980s, there were so many *unknowns* on the list dealing with exercise and reproduction that it became increasingly hard for anyone interested in the issue not to begin to study it. As a result, many groups began collecting information.

At about that time, my personal interest was rekindled by the results of an obstetrical resident's research project. This research indicated that, in Vermont, approximately 25 percent of women who were either currently pregnant or planning pregnancy engaged in regularly (three or more times each week) one or more types of sustained (20 minutes or more a session), strenuous (over 55 percent of their maximum intensity), weight-bearing exercise (Clapp and Dickstein 1984). Furthermore, over 90 percent of them planned to continue their exercise regimen during pregnancy. These numbers underscored the magnitude of the potential problem. If the ACOG was right—that sustained, vigorous exercise was harmful during pregnancy—then all concerned needed to know it quickly. If ACOG was wrong about exercise being harmful during pregnancy, then we needed to find out why they were wrong.

So, the next step was to recruit a small group of veteran recreational runners and aerobic dance instructors (who should have been at increased risk because of the high intensity and prolonged duration of their exercise sessions) before they conceived and compare the course and outcome of their pregnancies with those of a second, carefully matched control group of healthy, physically active, but nonexercising women. Using this approach we were able to study both sets of women and their babies before, during, and after their pregnancies, focusing on the interaction between the physiological changes produced by the exercise and those produced by the pregnancy. Our goal was not only to see what happened but also to understand why something did or did not happen at the same time.

The findings of the first study led to a second, then to a third, and so on. Now, some 10 years and well over 10 studies and 500 women later, I think we are beginning to understand what is going on (Clapp 1994a, 1996a).

The information provided by these studies and others is the subject of the remainder of this book. I hope that this historical perspective helps you clearly see the picture that emerges from the information presented later in the book and that it also helps you reach a conclusion regarding the place of recreational exercise and other forms of physical activity in the normal biology of reproduction. In the next chapter, we begin that journey with a discussion of the functional adaptations of a woman's body in response to regular exercise and in response to pregnancy, then try to predict what happens to the functional adaptations when the responses to exercise and those to pregnancy are combined.

Summary

I became interested in exercise during pregnancy over 20 years ago because many women chose to continue exercising during their pregnancies, yet we knew little about the effect it might have on the baby or the woman. Then as now, there were two schools of thought. The conservative school, which included most health care providers, felt that exercise during pregnancy was potentially harmful and therefore recommended a restrictive, cautious approach to exercise for healthy pregnant women. It sprang from the finding that a variety of maternal lifestyle factors could compromise pregnancy outcome and the knowledge that several physiological changes exercise induced could potentially harm a pregnancy.

The liberal school was represented by young women who had exercised regularly during one or more of their pregnancies. They felt that strenuous physical activity during pregnancy was not only normal but also helpful and recommended it to healthy women to improve the course and outcome of their pregnancies. This view had its origins in historical perspective and anecdotal or personal experience. These polarized views did two things. First, they generated conflict between active women, their health care providers, and often their friends and families as well. Second, they stimulated many different groups to begin to study the effects of exercise during pregnancy. We discuss many of these studies in the following chapter.

CHAPTER 2

Benefits of Exercising During Pregnancy

When I began these studies, I was in the same boat as everyone else. I was uncertain and needed additional information to decide whether exercise during pregnancy was a good idea, a bad idea, or didn't make any difference at all. On the one hand, physical activity was such an integral part of life that it was difficult to understand how it could be harmful to something as important as the reproductive process. On the other hand, it was equally difficult to understand why things like a sudden marked increase in temperature or a 50-percent decrease in blood flow to the womb would *not* harm the developing baby.

Because there were many theoretical concerns, little factual knowledge, and a growing number of women exercising vigorously during pregnancy, I decided it was time to study some veteran women competitive runners and aerobic dance instructors who maintained their exercise regimens throughout pregnancy. By studying these women, we would determine if the frequent (five or more times per week), prolonged (30 to 90 minute) bouts of high-intensity (65 to 90 percent of maximum capacity), weight-bearing exercise had any effect on the course and outcome of their pregnancies. Fortunately, our initial studies were designed to include objective measurements of many extra factors to avoid missing something important the first time around.

This approach required an immense amount of time and effort for everyone concerned, but it quickly paid off. When we began to analyze the information from the first 10 of these women, we were surprised and excited. Becoming pregnant had changed these women's bodily responses to their regular exercise routines! During very early pregnancy, their heart rates suddenly went sky-high, both at rest and during exercise (Clapp 1985b; Clapp and Capeless 1991a; Clapp, Seaward, et al. 1988). It was so early and dramatic that it alarmed several of the women, but it turned out to be simply an early, previously unrecognized sign of a healthy pregnancy. Later in the pregnancy, the heart rates of these women during exercise came back down. By late pregnancy, it was hard for most women to get their exercise heart rates up to the levels recorded before pregnancy, even though their workloads were the same or higher. Energy requirements during exercise also decreased, indicating that their metabolic efficiency had improved (Clapp 1989b), and suddenly their rectal temperatures were much lower at rest and during exercise (Clapp 1991; Clapp, Wesley, and Sleamaker 1987). Finally, during pregnancy, their blood sugar levels fell during and after exercise, which was the reverse of what happened before they became pregnant (Clapp and Capeless 1991a; Clapp, Wesley, and Sleamaker 1987).

These unexpected and dramatic changes were exciting because they meant that understanding the effects of exercise on the course and outcome of pregnancy might be straightforward. It looked as if many functional changes induced by the hormonal signals of pregnancy had modified various aspects of the exercise response in a manner that would protect the unborn baby. It also appeared that exercise-induced cardiovascular and metabolic training effects enhanced the functional changes of pregnancy in a manner that was also protective. Although this train of thought proved to be naive, it did provide a vital element of early understanding, helping us plan the experiments that eventually confirmed that very fit active women could maintain this level of physical activity throughout pregnancy without harm.

Over the next several years, we conducted many experiments to improve our understanding of the interaction between the changes induced by pregnancy and those induced by exercise. Eventually, we identified several critical factors at work in the interaction that led to an understanding of how regular, frequent (more than three times per week), sustained (20 minutes or more per session), moderate- to high-intensity, weight-bearing exercise influences the course and outcome of pregnancy for mother and baby. In turn, this enabled us to develop some rational principles to use as guidelines in designing holistic, individualized exercise programs for pregnant women.

Indeed, once the basic principles underlying the physiological inter-action between regular exercise and pregnancy are understood, it's easy to design an appropriate, individualized exercise regimen for any healthy woman who is either considering pregnancy or already pregnant. The remainder of this chapter is designed to start toward that goal. It will help you decide for yourself what is good about exercise during preg-nancy, what is bad about it, and what doesn't appear to make much difference at all.

The Heart and Circulatory System

Both pregnancy and exercise affect the function of a woman's heart and circulation at many levels and in many ways. The changes due to pregnancy are mediated by hormonal signals from the embryo, fetus, and placenta, and those due to exercise are induced by the stress of the increased function that exercise demands.

Adaptations to Pregnancy

During pregnancy, the entire circulatory system changes dramatically to support the needs of the woman's body and the increasing needs of her developing child (figure 2.1). Unfortunately, these changes also cause many of the unpleasant symptoms of pregnancy such as light-headedness, nausea, unbelievable fatigue, cravings, constipation, bloat-ing, frequent urination, and others. Even though these symptoms are disruptive, they are reassuring because their presence usually means a healthy pregnancy.

These adaptations actually begin very early, at or about the time the fertilized egg implants in the wall of the womb. The outer rim of cells destined to become the placenta initiate the changes by releasing hor-monal signals, which initiate relaxation and reduced responsiveness in most, if not all, the muscle cells in a woman's blood vessels (Duvekot et al. 1993; Hart et al. 1986). The result is that both the elasticity and volume of the entire circulatory system (heart, arteries, and veins) in-creases virtually overnight.

This creates a big problem: suddenly there is not enough blood in the circulation to fill it up. The amount of blood returning to the heart decreases as do the amount of blood in the heart and the amount the heart pumps out. As a result, blood pressure falls, especially when the preg-nant woman stands up. From the change in the amount of blood in the heart and the lower blood pressure, the body senses that the vascular

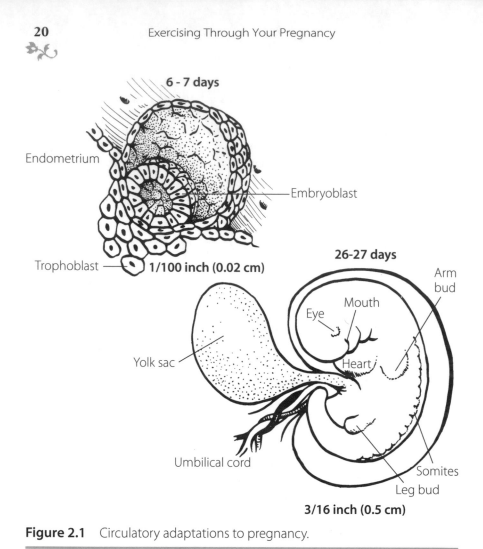

6 - 7 days

Endometrium

Embryoblast

Trophoblast — 1/100 inch (0.02 cm)

26-27 days

Arm bud

Mouth

Eye

Yolk sac

Heart

Umbilical cord

Somites

Leg bud

3/16 inch (0.5 cm)

Figure 2.1 Circulatory adaptations to pregnancy.

system is *underfilled*. In response, it triggers the release of several hormones from the heart and adrenal gland, which cause the body to decrease the excretion of salt and water by the kidneys. The retained extra salt and water rapidly expands the volume of plasma in the vascular system, correcting the underfill problem, and allows more blood to return to the heart so it can pump more out (cardiac output), thereby improving arterial pressure and blood flow to the organs. Eventually, the responses to the initial hormonal signals result in average increases in heart volumes (chamber volume and stroke volume, which is the amount of blood pumped with each beat) of 15 to 20 percent. Both blood volume and cardiac output increase by about 40 percent (Capeless and Clapp 1989; Clapp, Seaward, et al. 1988).

This all takes time, however. In the meantime, the woman may experience all the symptoms of vascular underfill that are usually present with either moderate dehydration or hemorrhage. These include the following:

- Waves of sudden fatigue
- A racing pulse
- Nausea
- Pallor
- Sweating
- Dizziness, especially when getting up quickly or during quiet standing

At first these symptoms are scary, but they improve progressively as the blood volume expands and usually are gone by the end of the fourth month.

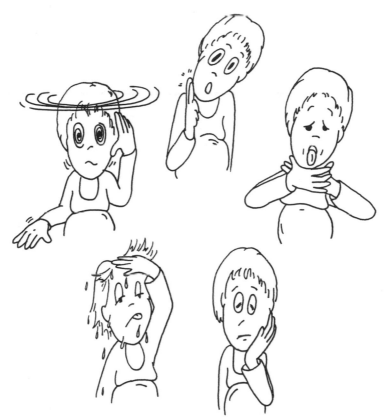

Wonders of early pregnancy.

The final circulatory adaptation to pregnancy is a blunted release of the stress hormones epinephrine and norepinephrine in response to a variety of stresses, including exercise (Clapp and Capeless 1991a). The blood vessels' responses to those hormones and similar drugs also are depressed (Nisell, Hjemdahl, and Linde 1985).

These adaptations eventually convert a relatively high-resistance, average-volume, normal–flow rate circulatory system into a low-resistance, high-volume, high-flow one needed to maintain the growth and development of the fetus within the body of the mother. The pressure in the arteries remains relatively low because the increase in the amount of blood pumped by the heart is still not great enough to match the degree of relaxation and dilation of the blood vessels that occurs. The vascular relaxation and dilation are most pronounced in the blood vessels that supply the skin, kidneys, and reproductive tissues. As a result, a large fraction of the additional blood available goes to these tissues, and their blood flows increase dramatically (2- to 20-fold) higher than before pregnancy.

These local changes in blood flow protect the baby but they also cause some bothersome symptoms for the pregnant woman. For example, the increase in skin blood flow raises skin temperature. While this improves a woman's ability to dissipate heat, it also makes her feel warm and appear flushed (especially in the palms and face). The increase in kidney blood flow improves waste removal, which ensures that the kidneys can handle the increased load of metabolic waste associated with the baby's growth. However, it also results in an increased volume of urine, which, along with pressure from the enlarging womb, stimulates frequent urination (a major problem for distance runners). Finally, the increased flow to the reproductive tissues ensures adequate delivery of oxygen and nutrients to the developing placenta and baby, but it also creates the uncomfortable sensation of pelvic and lower abdominal fullness.

Adaptations to Exercise

Many classic studies that identified the circulatory adaptations to exercise were done in the late 1960s and early 1970s (Saltin et al. 1968; Saltin and Rowell 1980). They clearly demonstrated that regular, vigorous exercise training increases blood volume, the size of the heart chambers, the volume of blood pumped with each beat, and the maximum cardiac output that can be achieved. It also increases the density and growth of blood vessels within skeletal muscle and the number of elements within the muscle cells that generate energy. In addition, it improves an individual's ability to dissipate heat by increasing the ability to sweat and lowering the temperature required to produce an increase in skin blood flow. These changes improve cardiovascular capacity, exercise capacity, and efficiency in many ways. For example, the need to shift blood flow away from the internal organs to the muscle during exercise is reduced, as are the heart rate, blood pressure, and thermal responses to any physical task. I'm sure you have noticed that five of these adaptations are similar to those induced by the hormonal signals of pregnancy. These include increases in the following:

- The volume of blood in the circulation
- The skin blood flow response
- The size of the heart chambers
- The volume of blood pumped each beat
- The delivery of oxygen to the tissues

Exercise increases blood volume, heart chamber volumes,
maximal cardiac output, blood vessel growth,
the ability to dissipate heat, and the delivery of oxygen
and nutrients to the tissues.

Interactive Effects

Therefore, as you might have already guessed, the changes produced by regular weight-bearing exercise actually complement those induced by pregnancy. Indeed, the circulatory status of a normal pregnant woman at rest has many similarities with that of a trained nonpregnant woman during exercise (volume expanded, hyperdynamic, high blood flows to tissue, and so on).

Moreover, it should be no surprise that when fit women maintain their exercise regimen during pregnancy, the cardiovascular adaptations to pregnancy are superimposed on their preexisting adaptations to training. The results of the interaction are at least additive. For example, the plasma volumes, red cell volumes, and total blood volumes of regularly exercising women during pregnancy are at least 10 to 15 percent higher than those of their sedentary sisters (Pivarnik et al. 1994). This means that women who exercise regularly during pregnancy have more circulatory reserve, which improves their ability to deal with both anticipated (exercise, work) and unanticipated circulatory stress (hemorrhage, trauma, anesthesia, and so forth). Likewise, in the active woman, pregnancy enhances the exercise-induced increases in left ventricular volumes. As a result, the amount of blood pumped by the heart each beat is 30 to 50 percent greater than that of a healthy but sedentary woman (Capeless and Clapp 1989; Robson et al. 1989).

When you combine the vascular adaptations to pregnancy with those to exercise, the effects are at least additive.

The only potential conflict between the circulatory demands of exercise and those of pregnancy is where the blood goes. During exercise it goes to supply the heart, muscles, skin, and adrenal glands, with a decrease in the flow to the renal, gastrointestinal, and reproductive systems. During pregnancy it goes to supply the reproductive tissues, kidneys, and skin, without significantly changing the rate of blood flow to other structures. From a safety point of view, the question is whether the cardiovascular adaptations in the fit, exercising, pregnant woman are sufficient to simultaneously maintain adequate blood flow and oxygen delivery to the exercising muscle and the fetus. As I discuss in later chapters, recent data indicates that, under most circumstances, the correct answer is the affirmative one (Clapp 1996a; Clapp, Little, et al. 1995).

Interpreting Exercise Heart Rates During Pregnancy

If you have ever wanted to prescribe or monitor exercise during pregnancy, you know that one of the most confusing areas is whether to use the heart rate response to exercise as a guideline. Before pregnancy, women who exercise regularly often use their heart rate response to exercise as a training intensity guide. To be sure that they are achieving a reasonable training effect from their exercise without risk, these women may determine their target heart rate range and work to keep their heart rate in this range. They determine their target heart range from a chart or calculate it as the range between 70 and 85 percent of their maximum heart rate (roughly calculated by subtracting their age from 220; American College of Sports Medicine 1994). So they quickly notice that their heart rate response to exercise changes during pregnancy and wonder why. Often, I've found the questions women ask about their heart rates express guarded concern and usually deal indirectly with issues of safety, health, or fitness. For example, the question, "Why does my heart rate go over 180 when I do aerobics?" really means, "Is it safe for the baby to let my heart rate go that high?" "Why does my heart race all the time?" means, "Do I have heart disease?" Finally, the question asked most often is "Do I really have to keep my heart rate under 140?" which means, "I don't feel like I'm getting a real workout; what can I do to maintain my fitness?"

The answer to each of these questions, as well as most others, is that it depends. Figure 2.2 details the possible reasons why heart rate is not a good predictor of how hard a woman is working during pregnancy and therefore is not a reliable measure of safety, health, or fitness. In fact, she probably is better off not monitoring it unless she knows a lot about her heart rate and its response to exercise before pregnancy. Indeed, it turns out that a pregnant woman's perception of how hard she is working using the Borg Rating of Perceived Exertion (RPE) scale may be a much better index of exercise intensity than her heart rate. Borg's scale allows the individual to numerically rate how hard she feels she is working, and it probably is the best way to monitor exercise intensity during pregnancy. I'll discuss how to use the Borg RPE scale in chapter 3.

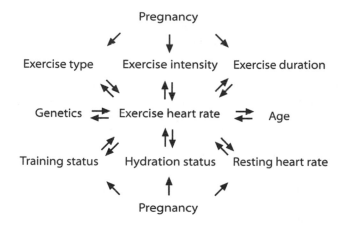

Figure 2.2   Factors altering heart rate.

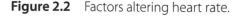

Pregnant or not, there are several reasons why relying solely on heart rate response during exercise is not the safest or most appropriate way to determine exercise intensity. Although there is a linear relationship between the intensity of exercise and the heart rate response in all individuals, the resting heart rate, slope of the heart rate response, maximum heart rate, environmental factors, and measurement technique vary from one individual to another. Some reasons you should not rely solely on heart rate response include the following:

1. A woman's genetic makeup can create a 15- to 30-beat per minute difference in her heart rate while exercising at a moderate to high intensity. Thus, individuals with low resting heart rates have lower heart rates at any exercise intensity, and vice versa.

2. A 20-year-old's exercise or target heart rate can easily be 10 to 20 beats per minute higher than a 35-year-old's at the same exercise intensity.

3. A person who trains regularly (unless she has overtrained) will have a lower heart rate at the same workload than one who does not.

4. When an individual is well hydrated, her exercise heart rate is lower than when she is behind on fluids, and late in an exercise session when plasma volume normally decreases the heart rate will be higher than at the beginning (this is what distance runners call *creep*).

5. The magnitude of the heart rate response to exercise is exercise-specific. It is greater during weight-bearing activity (running as opposed to biking or swimming) and when an individual uses more total muscle mass in the exercise or uses the arms vigorously (cross-country skiing or aerobics versus running).

6. Both resting and training heart rates vary with time of day, in relation to eating, anxiety, poor sleep, and so forth.

The superimposed effects of pregnancy on heart rate vary at different times in the pregnancy, making monitoring heart rate response even more confusing. During early pregnancy when the vessels are relaxed and dilated and the volume of blood has not yet caught up, resting heart rate will be elevated. Exercise heart rate at one's usual intensity will be extremely high because there is not enough blood in the system for the heart to pump the usual amount of blood each beat. Therefore it must pump more often to supply the same amount of blood to the exercising muscles. It's the same thing that happens when someone gets way behind on fluids. This pregnancy effect is so common that women who exercise regularly will often recognize they are pregnant because suddenly their exercise heart rate is sky-high and way out of proportion to how they feel.

As pregnancy proceeds, the blood volume rapidly expands to fill the dilated arteries and veins, and the amount of blood pumped by the heart each beat rises. However, resting cardiac output is going up, so resting heart rate does not come down, but exercise heart rate gradually falls. By midpregnancy, the relationship between heart rate and exercise intensity is usually similar to before conception. In late pregnancy, the combined effects of regular exercise and pregnancy appear to expand blood volume further. This probably increases the amount of blood the heart pumps each beat during exercise because, in the last 10 weeks of pregnancy, many fit women complain that they can't get their heart rate up to what they think it should be without working very, very hard.

Additional effects of pregnancy that influence the correct target or training heart rate include the changes in exercise parameters that influence overall training status. For example, a change from running to aerobics should increase the target heart rate, whereas a change from running to swimming should decrease it. The same is true for both the duration of each session (the longer the session, the higher the target heart rate needs to be) and how hard it feels (if it starts to feel easier at the usual heart rate, the target heart rate should be increased until it feels like it used to).

Thus, to assume you can use a standard target heart rate formula (such as 70 to 85 percent of age-predicted maximum heart rate) as a satisfactory guide for assessing the safety, health effects, and training effects of any exercise regimen during pregnancy seems unwise. During pregnancy, the exercise heart rate has value only when it is continuously monitored, interpreted in the context of pregnancy, and compared with serial measures that reflect exercise intensity and physiological effect (how hard it feels, oxygen consumption, fetal heart rate response, fatigue, and so on).

Now you see why I said "it depends." A heart rate of 180 or more— a racing heart—during high-impact aerobics in early pregnancy is normal for most women but would be unusual in a fit woman late in pregnancy. Likewise, an exercise heart rate of 130 to 140 during late pregnancy in a fit woman who trains five to seven hours a week is not uncommon when she is working in excess of 70 percent of her maximum capacity. In summary, no matter what her age or what stage she's at in pregnancy, how a pregnant woman feels before, during, and after a workout appears to be a better index of her health, safety, and quality of the workout than her heart rate response.

Lung and Placental Gas Transport

Pregnancy has several effects on lung function that improve the delivery of oxygen to the tissues of the mother and baby. In addition, a new organ develops in the wall of the womb (the placenta), which is structurally designed to maximize the efficiency of oxygen and carbon dioxide transfer between mother and baby. In contrast, exercise has no direct effect on the lung itself, but, by strengthening the muscles used in breathing, it does act indirectly to produce a small increase in maximum minute ventilation. It also improves the ability of tissues throughout the body to obtain and use the oxygen efficiently.

Adaptations to Pregnancy

Most aspects of lung function are improved by pregnancy. At rest the amount of air breathed increases by 40 to 50 percent or more because of an increase in the depth of each breath. This increase is the result of elevated levels of progesterone, which initiates *overbreathing* by increasing the sensitivity of the respiratory center in the brain to carbon dioxide. Although this is often associated with a feeling of breathlessness at rest or during mild exertion, it increases the oxygen tension and decreases the carbon dioxide tension in the tiny air sacs of the lung where gas exchange occurs. These directional changes in gas tension widen the pressure gradients, which improves the efficiency of oxygen uptake from the lung and the elimination of carbon dioxide from the blood and tissues of mother and baby. Although every pregnant woman feels that her capacity to breathe deeply is probably reduced, the elevation and widening of the rib cage during pregnancy actually improve it. Maximum breathing capacity is actually maintained at or above preconception levels (Artal, Fortunato, et al. 1995; DeSwiet 1991; Lotgering et al. 1991).

Beginning early in pregnancy, the increase in
progesterone stimulates breathing, which improves
the transfer of gases to and from the baby.
It also makes a woman feel
short of breath, but her lung function
remains normal.

The placenta, an organ unique to pregnancy, has many functions. One of these is to serve as the *fetal lung*. As such, the placenta is responsible for maintaining the transport of oxygen and carbon dioxide between mother and fetus. Like the lung, it possesses a variety of mechanisms that maintain oxygen delivery to the fetus under stressful circumstances. It has a large, highly vascularized surface that contains many extremely thin areas called vasculo-syncytial membranes, which improve the efficiency of gas transfer. Blood flows are high, and the vessel arrangement and blood flow directions in the two circulations maintain gas transfer when the maternal blood flow rate to the placenta falls by as much as 50 percent (figure 2.3). Differences in the type of hemoglobin in maternal and fetal red blood cells and the acidity of maternal and fetal blood also make gas transfer much more efficient. Subtle effects of exercise on any of these functional adaptations could either restrict or improve fetal oxygen availability.

Adaptations to Exercise

Changes in the blood flow distribution within the lungs during acute exercise improve the efficiency of gas transfer. However, we do not see long-term changes in most aspects of breathing and lung function in response to regular exercise or exercise training (Dempsey and Fregosi 1985; Hagberg, Yerg, and Seals 1988; Reuschlein et al. 1968). At a tissue and cellular level, the vascular and metabolic effects of regular exercise improve the body's ability to transport oxygen to the muscle cell during exercise. Exercise also improves the cell's ability to use that oxygen to perform work (Saltin et al. 1968; Saltin and Rowell 1980). It does the first by stimulating the growth of small new vessels in the muscle, which decreases the distance between vessels and between the muscles and the blood. This improves the availability of both oxygen and nutrients to the muscle cells and makes it easier for the cells to get rid of their metabolic wastes. The second thing exercise does is to increase the number of metabolism units, or *mitochondria*, in the cell, which allows the cell to produce energy from nutrients much faster. The combination of the two improves muscle strength and endurance.

Exercise does not improve lung function but improves gas transfer and oxygen availability and usage at the level of microcirculation and the cell.

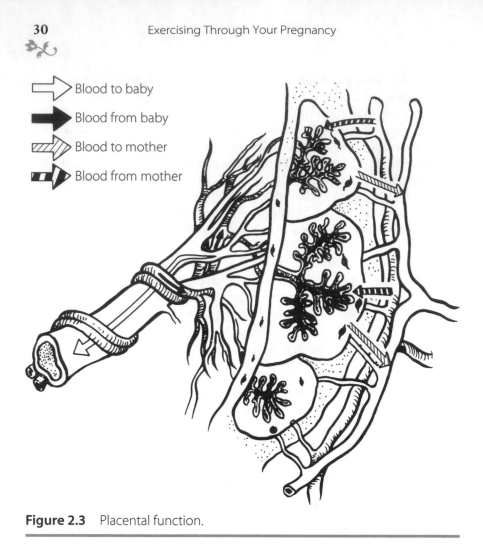

⇨ Blood to baby

⬛➡ Blood from baby

▨⇨ Blood to mother

▰➤ Blood from mother

Figure 2.3   Placental function.

There are two exceptions to the rule that regular exercise does not induce long-term changes in respiratory function. They are due to training effects on muscle, which we just discussed, that secondarily influence gas exchange and lung function. The result is that a trained individual has to breathe less air to get the same amount of oxygen during moderate exercise, and, during all-out exercise, maximal breathing capacity is increased.

Finally, I should point out that sustained exercise can acutely affect lung function in some otherwise normal individuals. In susceptible individuals, exercise can precipitate attacks of *exercise-induced asthma*, which appear to be due to smooth muscle constriction in the walls of the airways, responding to airway temperature and hydration changes. This constriction increases the resistance to air flow, which makes it difficult to breathe deeply and rapidly enough to meet the oxygen requirements for the exercise, so the athlete is forced to stop. The hormonal changes of pregnancy decrease the smooth muscle constriction, which improves the symptoms somewhat, but attacks still occur in susceptible individuals. Exercise-induced asthma is part of life for many athletes (Jackie Joyner-Kersee, for example) and is not a contraindication to exercise. It usually can be prevented by proper hydration and using one of several types of inhalers immediately before exercise.

Interactive Effects

Contrary to popular opinion, pregnancy does not compromise lung function during exercise in healthy, fit women. Indeed, because of the pregnancy-induced increase in alveolar ventilation, gas transfer at a tissue level should actually improve (Pivarnik et al. 1993; see also figure 2.4). Peak ventilation and absolute maximal aerobic capacity are maintained during pregnancy. It is probable that the combination of training and pregnancy improves maximal aerobic capacity by 5 to 10 percent (Clapp and Capeless 1991b; DeSwiet 1991; Lotgering et al. 1991). This *training effect* of pregnancy becomes most apparent six months to one year after the birth (Clapp and Capeless 1991b). It may explain the anecdotal reports of improved performance at national and international track and field events by women after having a baby. Likewise, the big increases in heart and blood volumes that occur by the 12th week of pregnancy should have the same effect as *blood doping*. This partially explains the outstanding performances of several female athletes from Eastern bloc countries who were at this stage of pregnancy when they competed in the 1976 Olympics.

> Pregnancy does not limit lung function, and both pregnancy and exercise improve the ability of body tissues to take up and utilize oxygen.

From the fetal point of view, the interactive effects of exercise and pregnancy adaptations on intrauterine oxygenation are both additive and protective (figure 2.5).

First, regular exercise during pregnancy has some unanticipated positive effects on the growth and function of the placenta that help to protect the fetus from oxygen deprivation. The placentas of women

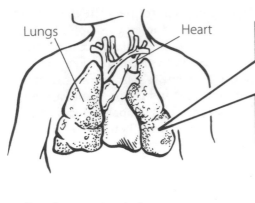

Lungs   Heart   Aveolus

Regular exercise during pregnancy
• induces an increase in aveolar ventilation,
• improves gas transfer at tissue level,
• maintains peak ventilation, and
• maintains absolute maximal aerobic capacity.
Pregnancy and exercise combined may improve $\dot{V}O_2$max by 5% to 10% six months to one year after the birth.

Figure 2.4   Lung adaptations to pregnancy and exercise.

who exercise regularly throughout early and midpregnancy grow faster and function better than those of women who are healthy but don't exercise regularly. This means that, at any rate of uterine blood flow, more oxygen and nutrients can get across to the baby of a woman who exercises than to the baby of one who does not. This probably is not important under most circumstances, because unless there is a problem or a large decrease in flow (as can occur with hemorrhage or strenuous exercise), both placentas will supply the baby adequately. When flow falls to low levels, however, the exercising woman's placenta can do a better job of maintaining fetal nutrition and oxygenation. I'll discuss this in greater detail in chapters 4 and 7.

Second, both exercise and pregnancy increase blood volume, and when the two are combined, the effect is additive. This extra increase in blood volume benefits and protects the fetus in the following ways.

• It makes it easier for the mother to maintain a higher blood flow rate to the placenta during exercise and other unanticipated events that can precipitously reduce the rate of uterine blood flow (hemorrhage, dehydration, anesthesia, and so forth).

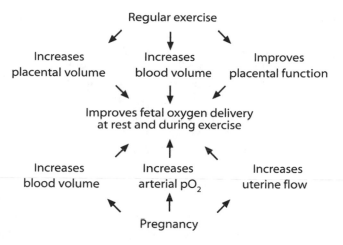

Figure 2.5   Factors affecting oxygenation.

- It may increase the rate of uterine blood flow under the circumstances of everyday life.
- Finally, the increased alveolar ventilation during pregnancy and the muscular effects of regular exercise on ventilation enhance placental gas transfer of oxygen and carbon dioxide between the mother and the baby.

Body Temperature and Sweating

Both pregnancy (a growth process) and regular exercise (mechanical work) generate extra heat that the mother's body must either store or eliminate. A woman's body responds to both thermal stresses by improving its capacity to eliminate the extra heat generated. The increase in weight and body tissue that accompanies pregnancy also improves a woman's capacity for heat storage. Indeed, at term, a pregnant woman can generate about 20 percent more heat without raising her body temperature because there is about 20 percent more tissue to keep warm.

Adaptations to Pregnancy

Maternal body temperature and many aspects of temperature regulation change dramatically during pregnancy. We know that increasing levels of progesterone cause a woman's basal temperature (measured first thing in the morning before getting up after a good night's sleep) to rise as much as 0.6 degrees centigrade (1.1 degrees Fahrenheit) in the last half of her menstrual cycle. If pregnancy ensues, it remains elevated for as much as the first 20 weeks of pregnancy. Therefore, we were surprised when we observed that body temperature actually fell during pregnancy once women were up and about for the day. We measured pregnant women's rectal temperature at standing rest for 10 minutes immediately before they began to exercise at their usual time. Starting very early in pregnancy, these women's resting body temperature fell dramatically and continued to fall progressively throughout the remainder of pregnancy (Clapp 1991). Not only did it fall as the pregnancy progressed, but, on each occasion, it fell progressively during the 10 minutes of quiet standing. This meant that, contrary to what we had thought, getting rid of excess heat generated by exercise was probably not going to be a problem for the women. Indeed, measurements of oxygen consumption under these circumstances suggested that their ability to get rid of heat had improved so much due to adaptations during pregnancy that the women had to increase their heat production to stay warm when they weren't active!

Pregnancy reduces the risk of a mother's temperature rising high enough to bother the baby by improving her ability to get rid of heat through her skin and lungs.

We discovered that two main factors cause this increase in the body's ability to dissipate heat.

1. Early in pregnancy, the body's set point for normal body temperature decreases. In earlier studies measuring basal body temperature, this finding was probably obscured by the increased metabolic heat generated by the growing fetus and placenta and the insulated environment under which the basal measurements were obtained (blankets and nighttime clothing).

2. The hormonal environment of pregnancy induces a marked increase in skin blood flow, which raises skin temperature on various parts of the body between two and six degrees centigrade (three and ten degrees Fahrenheit). It's this increase in blood flow that makes a pregnant woman's skin pink, which some people refer to as the *glow* of pregnancy. This change in skin temperature increases the rate of heat loss directly into the air around the woman. The so-called glow means

that she radiates a lot more heat to objects in her environment, warming them up, much like the sun does when it comes out from behind a cloud (Burt 1949; Katz and Sokal 1980).

Some other factors related to pregnant women being able to dissipate heat more rapidly include the following:

1. Pregnancy lowers the body's set point for sweating, which further improves the ability of the pregnant woman to get rid of heat once her core temperature starts to rise. During pregnancy, most women start to sweat as soon as their temperature rises. Because the skin is warm already, the sweat immediately evaporates, which extracts heat from their bodies, cooling them down.

2. The 40- to 50-percent increase in the amount of air a pregnant woman breathes improves ventilation and increases her ability to get rid of heat because the air she exhales is still at body temperature. So heat loss through breathing increases 40 to 50 percent as well.

3. The increases in blood volume and body weight or mass improve a pregnant woman's ability to deal with the extra heat. The increased blood volume maintains skin blood flow at high levels, which improves heat loss from the skin. The weight gain buffers any increase in heat production by progressively increasing the amount of tissue to heat by 5 to 10 percent in early pregnancy and by 20 to 25 percent near term.

We don't fully understand the mechanisms that induce these physiological changes, which improve a woman's ability to get rid of excess heat when she is pregnant, but they are probably hormonal in origin. For example, estrogen is known to increase skin blood flow and enhance heat storage capacity and heat loss in nonpregnant women by reducing resting core temperature and the thresholds for vasodilation and sweating (Stephenson and Kolka 1985; Tankersley et al. 1992). It is probable that it has the same effect during pregnancy.

Adaptations to Exercise

Regular sustained exercise alters at least two aspects of the thermoregulatory response to heat stress (Roberts et al. 1977; Saltin et al. 1968). As mentioned earlier, it increases blood volume, which improves an individual's ability to maintain skin blood flow at a high level during exercise, and it decreases the core temperature threshold for both cutaneous vasodilation and sweating (Roberts et al. 1977; Saltin et al. 1968). Both improve the capacity for heat dissipation in response to thermal stress.

Training improves a woman's ability to get rid of heat
by initiating dilation of the blood vessels in the skin
and sweating at a lower body temperature.

Interactive Effects

When a woman continues regular sustained exercise during pregnancy, the thermal adaptations to each complement one another, producing an additive positive effect (Clapp 1991) (figure 2.6). Thus, despite the theoretical concerns, a woman who exercises regularly can deal more effectively with heat stress when she is pregnant than when she is not. Her ability to dissipate heat and to store it increases during pregnancy. As a result, in early pregnancy her ability to tolerate heat stress improves by about 30 percent and in late pregnancy by at least 70 percent. Indeed, when a woman exercises at 65 percent of her maximum capacity in late pregnancy, her peak core temperature during exercise does not even get up to the level it was at rest before she became pregnant! This means that the risk of exercise inducing a significant increase in body temperature during pregnancy is extremely low unless the exercise is intense, prolonged, or conducted under extremely hot and humid conditions. Thus, with proper hydration and acceptable workout conditions, the issue of the baby's temperature rising too high during exercise may be a nonissue for all but the competitive athlete.

The effects of pregnancy and regular exercise, which improve
a woman's ability to get rid of excess heat, are additive.
As a result, a woman who exercises regularly can deal
more effectively with heat stress when she is
pregnant than a woman who does not exercise.

Metabolic and Hormonal Responses

The metabolic adjustments required for the growth and development of one new being within another are also regulated by a variety of hormonal

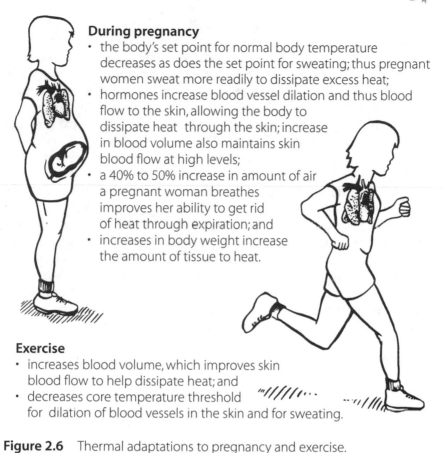

During pregnancy
- the body's set point for normal body temperature decreases as does the set point for sweating; thus pregnant women sweat more readily to dissipate excess heat;
- hormones increase blood vessel dilation and thus blood flow to the skin, allowing the body to dissipate heat through the skin; increase in blood volume also maintains skin blood flow at high levels;
- a 40% to 50% increase in amount of air a pregnant woman breathes improves her ability to get rid of heat through expiration; and
- increases in body weight increase the amount of tissue to heat.

Exercise
- increases blood volume, which improves skin blood flow to help dissipate heat; and
- decreases core temperature threshold for dilation of blood vessels in the skin and for sweating.

Figure 2.6 Thermal adaptations to pregnancy and exercise.

signals. These signals alter several traditional hormonal responses that influence the balance of nutrients (carbohydrate versus fat) the mother uses for fuel. Exercise training also changes the balance of nutrients used for fuel and the magnitude of the hormonal responses to physical stress.

Adaptations to Pregnancy

A major characteristic of pregnancy is that it is a growth process. With the formation of this new tissue, a pregnant woman's metabolic rate increases by 15 to 20 percent at rest, and she stores additional calories as well (Pernoll et al. 1975). In our society, much of the new tissue formed in early and midpregnancy is maternal fat (3 to 5 kilograms, or 7 to 11 pounds). As fat is rich in calories (9 kilocalories per gram), this represents the storage of 21,000 to 35,000 kilocalories. Feto-placental growth dominates late pregnancy and contributes about the same amount to maternal weight gain (3 to 5 kilograms, or 7 to 11 pounds; Clapp and Little 1995; Hytten 1991). However, these tissues contain less fat and thus have a lower caloric content per unit weight, representing only 9,000 to 15,000 kilocalories. The additional fluid retention and blood volume expansion of pregnancy have no calories but account for a fair amount of weight (4 to 7 kilograms, or 9 to 15 pounds). As a result, the pregnancy-associated weight gain for most women in western society averages 11 to 15 kilograms (24 to 33 pounds). However, the magnitude of each component (fat deposition, baby size, and fluid retention) is extremely variable between women in a single culture and between cultures. This suggests that the magnitude of each component is influenced by additional nongenetic factors, such as diet and activity (Clapp 1994b, 1997; King et al. 1994). For example, in third-world countries where women perform hard physical work and eat a marginal diet rich in complex carbohydrates and fiber, maternal weight gain is limited and fat deposition is minimal, but the baby's size is not much less than that in many industrialized societies.

> The metabolic changes occur to support the growth of the baby. They include fat deposition, changes in insulin sensitivity, and the suppression of stress responses and glucose release from the liver.

Another major metabolic change is a progressive increase in insulin resistance in maternal fat and muscle, which makes the pregnant woman's pattern of energy utilization similar to that of a mild diabetic. In mid- and late pregnancy, this change increases the amount of fat utilized to supply maternal energy requirements at rest and perhaps during exercise as well. From a fetal point of view, this change decreases maternal carbohydrate utilization (sugars), which makes it readily available for use by the fetus and placenta. As carbohydrate is normally their major source of energy, this change ensures an adequate nutrient supply for fetal and placental growth (Ryan, O'Sullivan, and Skyler 1985).

Pregnancy suppresses various aspects of the hormonal responses that increase the release of stored sugars from the liver when maternal blood sugar levels fall. It also prolongs the time it takes for food to travel through the intestines, which alters the absorption rate of nutrients into the blood. The combination of the two, coupled with the baby's increasing demand for sugar, leads to a rapid fall in maternal blood sugar levels if the woman goes for more than six to eight hours without eating.

Adaptations to Exercise

Regular exercise training does not consistently increase or decrease metabolic rate or body weight. It does, however, increase the maximal amount of energy a woman can generate and the amount of oxygen she can use each minute (maximum aerobic capacity or maximum work capacity) and alters the weight of the body's component parts (Saltin et al. 1968; Schultz et al. 1992; Stephanick 1993). In healthy reproductive-age women, regular weight-bearing exercise usually improves maximum aerobic capacity by about 20 percent and increases the weight of muscle and bone at the expense of fat. For example, if you examine two women who weigh 135 pounds, and one of them exercises regularly and the other does not, the one who exercises will be able to work much harder and likely have about 12 pounds, or 9 percent, less body fat. Over the years, that amount of body fat has been converted into muscle and bone by the regular exercise.

Exercise increases metabolic capacity, insulin sensitivity,
muscle mass, and the use of fat stores
to supply energy requirements.

Like pregnancy, regular exercise training increases the use of fat as an energy source at rest and during exercise. This spares sugar and maintains blood glucose levels at normal levels for a longer time during fasting or continuous exercise that would normally occur in nonexercising individuals (Coggan et al. 1990; Gollnick 1985). Unlike pregnancy, exercise training reduces insulin resistance, which allows the body to easily store sugar in its muscles after eating and during periods of rest. Finally, because training increases maximal aerobic capacity, it reduces the percentage of maximum capacity required to perform any task. This reduces the stress response to exercise (including the need to divert blood flow away from the internal organs to the muscles and the release of stress hormones).

Interactive Effects

In most respects, the metabolic changes induced by regular exercise and pregnancy complement one another (figure 2.7). The net effects are as follows:

- Increases maternal reliance on fat for energy, which improves the availability of glucose and oxygen for the fetus and placenta
- Suppresses the hormonal and circulatory aspects of the stress response, which minimizes the decrease in uterine blood flow during exercise

However, the suppression of glucose release from the liver during pregnancy, coupled with the increased insulin sensitivity that regular exercise produces, decreases the glucose available for the baby during exercise and possibly at rest if food intake is sporadic. For this reason, in part III, I discuss in more detail what and when a pregnant woman who exercises regularly should eat.

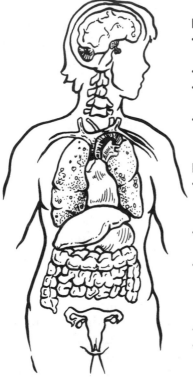

Pregnancy
- increases mother's metabolic rate by 15% to 20% at rest,
- increases mother's ability to store calories,
- progressively increases insulin resistance in maternal fat and muscle, and
- increases use of fat as energy in late pregnancy (and sparing sugar for baby).

Regular exercise
- increases maximal amount of energy a woman can generate and the amount of oxygen she can use each minute,
- alters the weight of the body's component parts,
- increases use of fat as an energy source at rest and during exercise (sparing sugar and maintaining more constant blood glucose levels),
- reduces insulin resistance, and
- reduces stress response to exercise.

Figure 2.7   Metabolic and hormonal adaptations to pregnancy and exercise.

Combining regular exercise with pregnancy
improves the supply of glucose and oxygen for the baby
under most circumstances *if* the mother-to-be
eats adequately and regularly.

Muscle, Ligament, and Bone Adaptations

Both pregnancy and regular exercise have a variety of effects on muscle, ligament, and bone. The effects of pregnancy have not been explored in detail, but the effects of exercise have been thoroughly studied.

Adaptations to Pregnancy

Unfortunately, the pregnancy-associated functional changes in muscle, ligament, and bone have not received the attention they deserve. Clearly, the increase in a woman's weight (often 15 to 25 percent of her prepregnancy weight) and the enlarging abdomen increase mechanical stress on the back, pelvis, hips, and legs. The change in a woman's center of gravity (up and out) and the stretching and loosening of the ligaments that stabilize the pelvis, hips, and low back decrease mobility and increase musculoskeletal stress (Abramson, Robert, and Wilson 1934; Ellis, Seedhom, and Wright 1985). Given these changes, it is amazing that musculoskeletal complaints and injuries are not more common. The only common musculoskeletal complaint related to these changes is low-back pain (Berg et al. 1988; Östgaard et al. 1994).

During pregnancy bone density is maintained
and ligaments relax. Changes in muscle function
are unclear, warranting further study.

Several laboratories have examined calcium balance and changes in bone density during pregnancy (Heaney and Skillman 1971; Sowers et al. 1991). Although limited, their findings are reassuring. It appears that bone mineral is maintained even though bone turnover increases.

One reason for this may be that the intestinal absorption of calcium becomes more efficient during pregnancy.

What happens during pregnancy to ligamentous support and tension in the head, neck, shoulders, and peripheral joints is controversial. Most assume that the ligamentous laxity in the pelvis (hips and lumbosacral spine) is present throughout the body. Evidence to support this has been provided for many joints but only when significant external force is applied (Calganeri, Bird, and Wright 1982; Schauberger et al. 1996). In any case, any changes that do occur do not impair joint function or increase the risk of injury (Karzel and Friedman 1991; Schauberger et al. 1996).

No one has looked at whether muscle mass or muscle function (the force and velocity of contraction) changes during pregnancy. However, several observations suggest that both muscle mass and strength increase. First, in the only study in which it has been measured, lean body mass after pregnancy was about five percent greater than before pregnancy (Little, Clapp, and Ridzon 1995). As bone mineral is unchanged, the difference is probably due to an increase in muscle mass. Second, the fact that a woman carries around an additional 20 or more pounds during late pregnancy should increase muscle size and strength in the lower extremities. Results from an earlier study, however, indicate that women do not maintain this mass and strength long-term. Lean body mass was unchanged from preconception values one year postpartum in a group of 10 women runners (Clapp and Capeless 1991b). But these women's postpartum training never got back to their preconception levels.

Adaptations to Exercise

Numerous studies have documented that regular exercise training has many positive effects on muscle, ligament, and bone. It increases muscle mass and the force and velocity of contraction as well as improving coordination. The mechanical stresses of training also improve ligamentous tensile strength and bone density. However, these effects are site-specific, meaning that they are a response to stress and therefore dependent on the individual's specific training program (Drinkwater et al. 1984; Gollnick et al. 1981; Henriksson 1977; Saltin and Rowell 1980; Tipton, Vailas, and Matthes 1986). The marked difference in strength between the muscles of the upper and lower extremity in fit women who do not weight train or do lots of other upper body work is a classic example.

---

*Regular exercise improves most, if not all,
aspects of musculoskeletal function, and its effect on bone
is enhanced by ovarian hormones.*

Finally, a woman's ovarian hormones (estrogen and progesterone) enhance the effects of exercise on bone as they positively affect bone turnover, remodeling, and density. The osteopenic effects of amenorrhea, menopause, and lactation on bone density and the preventive value of estrogen replacement therapy emphasize the important role these hormones play in maintaining or increasing bone mineral content and density. The specific role of progesterone alone in bone turnover and remodeling remains controversial, however, as not all investigators have been able to demonstrate that it has a clear-cut effect (Clapp and Little 1995).

Interactive Effects

Theoretically, the effects of exercise should either counterbalance or enhance the effects of pregnancy on muscle mass and strength. However, our laboratory has not seen any additive effect of regular exercise on the increase in lean body mass that normally occurs in healthy, physically active women during pregnancy (Little, Clapp, and Ridzon 1995). Likewise, one would think that the high levels of estrogen and progesterone, coupled with the continued mechanical stresses of exercise, should enhance bone remodeling and increase bone density. But at least two groups have shown no clear overall additive effect of exercise and pregnancy on bone density. Furthermore, their data suggest that if there is any additive effect it may be site-specific and vary with the stage of the pregnancy and the type of exercise (Drinkwater and Chestnut 1991; Little, Clapp, and Gott 1993).

Regular exercise should offset the effects of pregnancy on ligamentous laxity, improve strength, maintain muscle tone, and reduce the incidence of low-back pain and other musculoskeletal complaints. It should also minimize the inevitable upward and outward shift in a woman's center of gravity as her uterus grows and protrudes, by maintaining back strength, good posture, and abdominal muscle tone. Data from our laboratory and those of others dealing with exercise-associated injuries, physical symptomatology, physical efficiency, maximum aerobic capacity, pregnancy weight gain, and subcutaneous fat deposition support this conclusion (Clapp 1989b, 1996a; Clapp and Capeless 1991b; Clapp and Little 1995; Östgaard et al. 1994; Wallace et al. 1986).

Summary

The medical and safety issues about exercise during pregnancy are based on the concern that high body temperature, reduced delivery of oxygen and nutrients to the placenta and baby, mechanical stress, and trauma may result in damage to baby or mother. However, the physiological effects of combining exercise and pregnancy are different than anticipated and do not support these concerns. The reason is that the functional changes from exercise either compensate for or complement the functional changes of pregnancy, and vice versa. Therefore, the combination produces physiological change that creates an extended margin of safety for both mother and baby under conditions of cardiovascular, metabolic, thermal, and mechanical stress. As such, these adaptations would protect both should unanticipated medical problems arise in late pregnancy, labor, or delivery.

In terms of exercise stress, the changes in blood volume and vascular reactivity maintain blood flow to the placenta. The changes in ventilation and placental development combine with the metabolism changes to improve the availability of oxygen and energy-producing sugar for the baby's growth without compromising maternal function. Likewise, the improved ability to dissipate heat protects against thermal injury, and the musculoskeletal and ligamentous effects of regular exercise protect the mother from significant symptomatology or injury.

The $64,000 question is "Are these interpretations right?" Part II describes our experience in attempting to answer this question.

PART II

How Exercise Benefits Mother and Baby

This part of the book is a *must-read* for relatives of expectant mothers, because it is full of pleasant surprises that should alleviate their concerns. Its purpose is to present the new factual information we and others have gathered about exercise in pregnancy in order that the reader may decide if our interpretation (that combining regular exercise with pregnancy is beneficial for both mother and baby) is right or not. In addition, the information it contains is the basis for the approach to exercise prescription I recommend in part III.

These next five chapters detail the impact of regular weight-bearing exercise on many aspects of the course and outcome of pregnancy, breast-feeding, and the growth and development of the baby after birth. In doing so, these chapters provide unbiased factual information that helps to answer most, if not all, of the questions and concerns voiced by both the women we have studied and their health care providers.

Specifically, chapter 3 focuses on the issues surrounding and findings about the impact of exercise on fertility, miscarriage, and congenital defects. Chapter 4 examines the controversies as well as the findings of the relationships among physical stress, recreational exercise, premature birth, and fetal growth retardation. Chapter 5 looks at the relationships among regular exercise after the birth, lactation performance, infant growth, and maternal weight loss. Chapters 6 and 7 detail the multiple benefits of regular exercise during pregnancy that we have identified for both the mothers and their offspring. Specific maternal topics discussed include the following: weight gain and fat deposition, discomfort and injury, medical complications, course and outcome of labor and delivery, fitness, performance, and what happens after the birth. Chapter 7 focuses on the following: the normal and abnormal fetal responses to maternal exercise, fetal well-being, fetal responses to labor, condition at birth, why babies benefit from maternal exercise, and postnatal growth and development in the first five years of life. Watch out, it contains lots of surprises!

CHAPTER 3

Exercise, Fertility, and Early Pregnancy

This chapter discusses the discrepancies between the medical and safety concerns and the observed reproductive outcomes in exercising women. The chapter aims to provide you with the information you need to answer two questions that bother many exercising women, trainers, and health care providers:

1. Does regular, sustained exercise decrease the ability of a woman to conceive?
2. Does continuing regular, sustained exercise into pregnancy cause other troubles in the first three months of pregnancy?

The Confounder Issue

Before we answer these questions, it is important to understand the influence of what I call the *confounder* issue. It's amazing, but when a woman has a history of regular exercise, it influences others' attitudes about her reproductive capacity. Indeed, such a history typically produces a knee-jerk response from some health care providers who have stereotypical ideas of what being an athletic woman is all about, which inevitably alters, or *confounds*, their approach to diagnosis and therapy. The stereotype often includes three specific attributes that some feel have detrimental effects on fertility and the course and outcome of pregnancy. These assumed attributes of regularly exercising women are as follows:

1. They are underweight and do not have a normal amount of body fat.
2. They don't eat enough calories.
3. Their time commitment to exercise creates both physical and emotional stress.

These three misconceptions deserve discussion because, although they are commonly held, they don't apply to most athletic women. The first (athletic women are all underweight and too skinny) is usually interpreted as indicating abnormal reproductive function. This stereotypic view arose from earlier studies of women with eating disorders, which suggested that a woman's body fat needed to be more than 18 to 21 percent for normal menstrual and ovarian function (Frisch and MacArthur 1974). Unfortunately, the fact that the women in these early studies were not necessarily athletic is usually forgotten, and, by inference, this led to the idea that all lean, athletic women have abnormal menstrual cycles and have difficulty conceiving. Likewise, there is a crude relationship between a woman's prepregnancy weight and both the size of the baby at birth and several complications of pregnancy. So, again by inference, light, athletic women should be at risk for several late-pregnancy complications, including a low birth weight baby.

However, the suggestion that a lower percent body fat alone interferes with menstrual function, ovulation, and ability to conceive is incorrect (Clapp 1994a; Sanborn, Albrecht, and Wagner 1987; Warren 1980). Likewise, the effect of prepregnancy weight on birth weight and pregnancy complications in well nourished women is minimal except when weight per unit height is very low (Hunscher and Tompkins 1970). Thus, the average woman who exercises regularly does not increase her chance of difficulty because of either her weight or her percent body fat (Clapp 1994a). Nonetheless, many health care providers still feel that lean, light, physically active women have an increased incidence of ovulatory disorders causing infertility and a greater chance of delivering a low birth weight baby.

The second stereotypic attribute (athletic women eat like birds) is interpreted to mean that they are either malnourished or have an eating disorder. As both malnourishment and eating disorders are associated with ovulatory and menstrual abnormalities and poor pregnancy outcome (King et al. 1994; Marshall 1994), then, by inference, athletic women should be at increased risk. This risk may be true for some women with additional risk factors (Loucks et al. 1992; Marshall 1994). However, most noncompetitive, healthy women who exercise have dietary habits well above average in the quantity and quality of their caloric intake and nutrient mix (Clapp and Little 1995).

Many health care providers mistakenly believe that most women who exercise experience abnormal reproductive function because they are *underweight, malnourished,* and *stressed-out.*

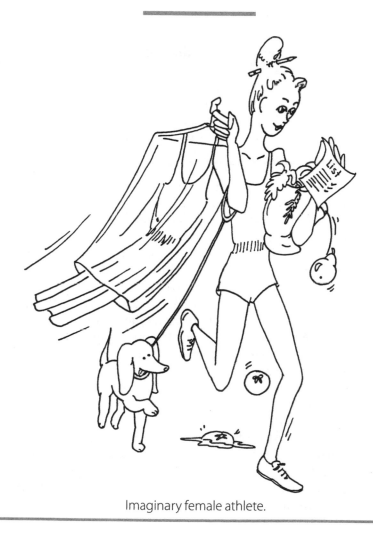

Imaginary female athlete.

The third stereotypic attribute (athletic women are stressed-out and under pressure all the time), is also interpreted as a "red flag," indicating disordered reproductive function because excessive physical or emotional stress is known to suppress ovarian function (Marshall 1994). That may be the case in some national class athletes or in disciplines as demanding as gymnastics and ballet. Most women who exercise recreationally, however, view their exercise as a stress reliever rather than a stress generator. Indeed, most athletic women vigorously protect their time spent exercising because they view it as valuable personal relaxation time in an otherwise busy, overcommitted life.

Fertility Issues

There are several reasons why questions about the effects of regular, strenuous exercise on fertility have not been clearly answered long before this. First, infertility is common (affecting 5 to 10 percent of couples) and so is exercising (10 to 25 percent of married, reproductive-age women exercise). Thus, purely by chance, many women who have difficulty becoming pregnant will also exercise regularly. Again, this creates the problem of guilt by association, which often confounds the approach to diagnosis and therapy. For example, if it is either difficult or prohibitively expensive to find the cause for infertility, then a physician may use lifestyle factors to help explain the unexplainable. For many women who exercise regularly and have difficulty conceiving, this translates into, "I can't find anything to explain why you can't get pregnant; perhaps if you cut back on your exercise and gain a little weight, it will solve the problem." All too often this means a year goes by before additional diagnostic steps are taken.

Another explanation is that no one looked seriously at the question of the effect of exercise on fertility because the prevailing opinion had been that exercise and athletics do contribute to infertility in women. In the 1980s, this long-standing opinion received scientific support from the results of two studies. They documented that exercise can suppress or alter the normal patterns of hormonal secretion that regulate the production and release of eggs from the ovary (Bullen et al. 1985; Loucks et al. 1989). Although these results were clear, the training program in the first study (Bullen et al. 1985) was atypical (sudden onset of high-volume training in untrained women). In the second (Loucks et al. 1989), marginal nutritional intakes and life stressors other than exercise may have contributed. Finally, neither directly tested the issue of fertility in the women studied.

Fertility of Regular Exercisers

When we began our studies of exercise during pregnancy we specifically asked these questions:

- Were these studies right?
- Do women who exercise regularly have more trouble getting pregnant when they want to than those who don't?

To answer these questions and those that follow, we enrolled more than 250 pairs of healthy, physically active women planning pregnancy before they tried to get pregnant. About 60 percent of these women were planning their first pregnancy, and none of these had a history of miscarriage or trying unsuccessfully to get pregnant. The remainder were planning either their second or third pregnancy and, to avoid bias, those with a history of miscarriage or diseases which might result in infertility were excluded from this part of the study.

The only difference between the two women comprising each of the pairs was that one of the women regularly engaged in sustained, weight-bearing exercise (mostly aerobics and running), and the other did not. Most of those who exercised were strictly *recreational athletes* (that is, they exercised continuously for 20 to 60 minutes three to five times a week; only 15 percent of these exercisers either taught aerobics classes or competed more than three times a year). However, the between-individual range in exercise performance was broad. The time spent in each session ranged from 20 to 135 minutes, with a mean of 47 minutes. Individual exercise intensities required between 51 and 90 percent of the individual's maximum oxygen consumption (maximum aerobic capacity) with a group average of 64 percent. For most individuals, this intensity of exercise was perceived as moderately hard to very, very hard equating to between 14 and 18 on the Borg Rating of Perceived Exertion (RPE) scale (see figure 3.2) and produced a rise in pulse rate to between 145 and 190 beats per minute. The number of exercise sessions a week ranged between 3 and 11, with a modal value of 4 for the group.

Our approach was simple. We chose a strict definition of infertility (inability to get pregnant within six months) and kept track of the exercise and how long it took the women to get pregnant once they were ready. Then we compared the rate of infertility in the two groups.

Most healthy women can exercise vigorously
without interfering with their fertility.

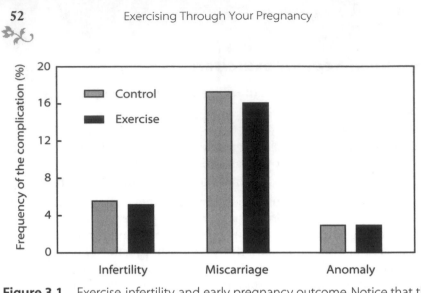

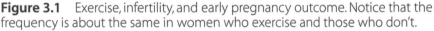

Figure 3.1   Exercise, infertility, and early pregnancy outcome. Notice that the frequency is about the same in women who exercise and those who don't.

Figure 3.1 illustrates the findings. Exercise at these levels didn't make any difference one way or the other! The incidence of infertility was between five and six percent in the women who exercised and in the physically active controls. Furthermore, although the numbers of women with exceptionally high exercise performance are still small, we have been unable to detect either a dose-response or a threshold effect for infertility within this group, most of whom exercise because it's fun and makes them feel good. Thus, although exercise can interfere with normal ovulatory and menstrual function, when we look at fertility prospectively in women without a history of fertility problems, we cannot detect an effect over a wide range of exercise performance.

In my view, this means that most healthy women can obtain many of the physiological benefits of exercise without it interfering with fertility. Weight-bearing exercise for 20 minutes or more, three or more times a week, at an intensity that feels moderately hard to hard (this usually equals or exceeds 55 percent of an individual's maximal aerobic capacity) is enough. This equals a rating of 14 to 15 on Borg's 6 to 20 scale of perceived exertion. We have reproduced this scale in figure 3.2 (Borg 1998). It's a handy training tool that is much easier and more accurate than measuring heart rate, especially during pregnancy. It's based on the logical principle that how an individual feels is an accurate indicator of how hard she is working relative to her maximum capacity. For example, a rating of "6" is how you feel when you are in bed, an "11" is how most active people feel when they walk, a "20" is when you think you are going to pass out from exertion.

6	No exertion at all
7	
8	Extremely light
9	Very light
10	
11	Light
12	
13	Somewhat hard
14	
15	Hard (heavy)
16	
17	Very hard
18	
19	Extremely hard
20	Maximal exertion

Figure 3.2   Borg's Rating of Perceived Exertion (RPE) scale.

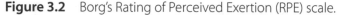

If you want more fitness and performance benefits (which are dose-response effects), you can do a lot more than the minimum required for basic fitness without interfering with your fertility. However, a word of caution is in order. These recommendations come from experience with a specific group of women and a specific range of exercise performance; thus, the same may not be true for all types of exercise or for all women. I suspect that there is a threshold level of exercise above which infertility does become a problem. Although it is high, it can probably be lowered by stress from other sources (nutrition, work, interpersonal difficulties, and so on). Thus, infertility may be a problem for many women when they perform at much higher training levels, such as those required for athletes who compete at the collegiate or national level. The same is probably the case for exercising women who have preexisting ovulatory disturbances or other organic (e.g., tubal obstruction) or psychiatric disease (e.g., anorexia nervosa).

The Fertility of Nonexercisers

The important question for this group of women is "Should a woman begin an exercise program at the same time she is trying to become pregnant?" Unfortunately, there is no information available for the types of programs that previously sedentary women usually enroll in to improve fitness (brisk walking, aerobics, cycle ergometry, stair climbers, and the like). The information from one training study, which started women on a very intensive training program (Bullen et al. 1985), however, suggests that if you don't regularly exercise, *starting an intense training program* should be avoided while trying to conceive because it acutely alters menstrual patterns and presumably ovulation as well. Nonetheless, without information to the contrary, it seems that most low-intensity programs (perceived difficulty only slightly to moderately hard, 12 to 14 on Borg's RPE scale) that initially limit sustained endurance training to 20 minutes or less and that emphasize developing flexibility (lots of stretching) are fine because the physical stress level is relatively low.

Early Pregnancy Issues

The concern is that exercise-associated changes, such as increased body temperature, decreased uterine blood flow, changes in hormonal levels, and mechanical stresses from jumping or running, will cause things like ectopic or tubal pregnancy (a pregnancy developing outside the womb); spontaneous abortion (miscarriage); defects in the developing baby; or abnormal development of the placenta to occur more frequently. But there have been no reports confirming these concerns.

Therefore, when we began our studies we asked "If women continue to exercise at their prepregnancy levels throughout early pregnancy, will it increase the frequency of these complications?" To answer this question, we continued following the remaining pairs of women throughout pregnancy. We also *added* more than 80 matched pairs who did not qualify for the initial fertility study because of a history of abortion or other reproductive difficulties.

Miscarriage and Congenital Defects

Spontaneous miscarriage often follows conception and is another area in which guilt by association can be a problem for regularly exercising women who become pregnant. It occurs so frequently that it is not considered abnormal unless a woman has three in a row. How common it is depends on the overall health of the women studied and how hard you look for it. In the women we studied, we expected that a *normal* rate would be somewhere between 15 and 20 percent. This meant we would have to be careful in our diagnosis of both pregnancy and miscarriage in all the women to avoid the guilt by association problem because the exercising women were much more concerned about it and often ran their own pregnancy tests at home. Therefore, we took great pains (very early pregnancy test and ultrasound exam) to be sure that we identified and categorized all cases of spontaneous miscarriage correctly.

Continuing regular, vigorous exercise throughout
early pregnancy *does not* increase the incidence
of either miscarriage or birth defects.

As illustrated in figure 3.1, continuing regular aerobics or running throughout early pregnancy does not increase or decrease the incidence of spontaneous abortion or miscarriage. This rate has remained 16 to 17 percent in both groups (exercisers and nonexercisers) for the last six years (Clapp 1989a, 1994a). Reports from retrospective questionnaire studies of pregnant runners also indicate that the rate of spontaneous miscarriage is not increased by running in early pregnancy (Cohen et al. 1989; Jarrett and Spellacy 1984; Melpomene Institute and USMS Sports Medicine Research Committee 1989).

Likewise, regular weight-bearing exercise throughout early pregnancy has not increased the incidence of congenital malformation, which has remained between two and three percent in both groups. This rate is also the incidence in the general population. Although this low incidence means we would have to study several thousand women to be sure, it appears that continuing regular exercise throughout early pregnancy does not increase the chance of a birth defect in the baby. Moreover, the fact that we have been unable to demonstrate a difference supports the conclusion that the pregnancy-associated improvement in the ability to dissipate heat has made thermal stress and subsequent malformation a nonissue under usual conditions for most women who choose to maintain their exercise regimen during early pregnancy.

Ectopic Pregnancy and Other Placental Problems

Much to our surprise, to date we have encountered only one case of ectopic or tubal pregnancy in the more than 500 women who have enrolled in either the exercise or control group. This is unusual because the frequency of this complication is rising in the population at large. Perhaps it is because none of the women we studied smoke, and none have had a history of pelvic infection. Most are monogamous and have a stable lifestyle. All three of these factors (smoking, pelvic inflammation, and sexual practices) have been implicated in the increasing incidence of ectopic pregnancy.

In any case, the incidence of ectopic pregnancy is not increased in women who continue to exercise at or above a level that provides them with many fitness benefits (minimum of 20 minutes, three times a week, at a perceived intensity that is moderately hard to hard). As a matter of fact, it looks as if a woman's exercise habits are unrelated to ectopic pregnancy.

Finally, we have seen no suggestion that continuing regular exercise at these levels increases the incidence of other diseases related to abnormalities in placental growth and development. Specifically, this includes the placenta implanting right inside the mouth of the womb (placenta previa), the placenta separating from the wall of the womb before the baby is born (placental abruption), poor placental growth or lots of placental damage, and the onset of high blood pressure during pregnancy (pregnancy-induced hypertension). As with the birth defects issue, however, the numbers are a problem. The frequency of each complication is very low in both groups and in the population at large, so we can't be absolutely sure whether regular exercise in early pregnancy contributes to or prevents one or more of these complications unless we study thousands of women. Still, we can be sure that if there is an effect, it is quite small—or we would have seen a trend by now.

So, it appears that women can continue their regular exercise regimen and maintain or improve their fitness level throughout early pregnancy without increasing their chances of miscarriage, birth defects, or placental disease. The range of exercise performance we have encountered has been large, and, within the limits discussed, it appears that more than the minimum exercise required for basic fitness (20 minutes, three times a week, at a moderately hard to hard level of effort) should provide more benefit without increasing risk.

Summary

Concerns about the safety of exercise while attempting pregnancy and during early pregnancy initially arose, then were supported by interpreting anecdotal information and scientific results out of context. These concerns have been self-perpetuated by some health care providers who view the female recreational athlete as suffering from exercise-induced problems she doesn't have. Despite these beliefs, there is no evidence in our studies or those of others that healthy women need to change their exercise habits when they plan to conceive or during early pregnancy in order to get pregnant easily or reduce their risk of miscarriage, tubal pregnancy, birth defect, or placental disease. Beginning an exercise program at this time is unstudied, but it appears that it should be safe as long as the effort expended is limited to a rating of 12 to 14 on the Borg RPE scale (<60% of $\dot{V}O_2$max) and the duration of each session is limited to 20 to 30 minutes.

CHAPTER 4

Exercise, Premature Labor, and Feto-Placental Growth

This chapter focuses on the discrepancy between the theoretical concerns that exercise during mid- and late pregnancy will initiate labor or restrict fetal growth and the actual outcomes observed. It provides information that answers the following questions exercising women often ask in the latter half of their pregnancies:

- If I continue to exercise, will I deliver early?
- I get cramps when I exercise, does that mean I'm ready to go into labor?
- Some people are surprised when they find out I'm already six months pregnant; is my baby too small?
- Why does my sister show more than I do when I'm further along?
- I'm much smaller this pregnancy and feel great; is it because I'm exercising this time?

I begin with some background information on physical stress and focus on an important underlying mechanism linking physical stress and pregnancy complications. Then I cover the findings on recreational exercisers. Although the effects are much different, I mention both because I feel the lesson learned from the physical stress story is valuable and can be applied when designing an individualized exercise program for use in pregnancy.

Physical Stress, Fetal Growth, and Pregnancy Length

The concerns that exercise might initiate labor early or restrict the growth of the baby come from two unfounded sources. First, there is an unsubstantiated concern that the recurrent, exercise-associated decreases in uterine blood flow and blood sugar levels, coupled with the increase in stress hormones, may initiate uterine contractions ahead of schedule or deprive the baby of necessary nutrients. The second concern, which reinforces the first, comes from research in industrial medicine indicating that several types of on-the-job physical stress increase the incidence of labor starting more than three weeks before the baby is due (so-called premature labor). The research also shows that these stresses increase the number of infants who weigh less than they should for the time they are born (Luke et al. 1995; Mamelle, Laumon, and Lazar 1984; Naeye and Peters 1982). Furthermore, intervention trials have clearly demonstrated that reducing physical stress in the workplace eliminates these two problems (Huel et al. 1989). Faced with these findings, many reasoned that physical stress is physical stress no matter where you find it. As a result, it was assumed that vigorous recreational activities would produce the same effect and should be avoided (another example of a pregnant woman experiencing guilt by association).

However, the types of physical stress in the workplace that have had significant effects are much different physiologically from those of recreational exercise. These work-related physical stresses include

- quiet standing for four or more hours a shift,
- walking for protracted periods,
- long work shifts, and
- frequent heavy lifting.

The combined effects inevitably produce feelings of extreme fatigue in a pregnant woman. When a woman experiences this fatigue regularly at the end of her shift, it appears to be a valuable warning sign indicating that her risk of delivering an undergrown baby prematurely is high unless changes are made in her job requirements. Indeed, some investigators (Luke et al. 1995) have developed a job *fatigue index score* that can be used for any working pregnant woman to assess her job-related risk for both premature labor and a smaller than average baby.

The fact that these stresses produce symptoms of extreme fatigue well before either premature labor or the growth rate of the baby actually slows makes good physiological sense. The symptoms of extreme fatigue in any healthy person (pregnant or not) usually reflect severe dehydration and nutrient depletion. When it occurs in a pregnant woman after four or more hours of quiet standing or a long, busy shift, it likely reflects the same thing. Although the overall sequence of events (busy job, quiet standing, dehydration, extreme fatigue) has not actually been studied, it probably goes like this:

1. The woman has been busy or is allowed infrequent breaks so she doesn't drink because she doesn't have time.
2. If she can drink, she doesn't because it will mean many trips to the ladies' room.
3. This dehydration is compounded by her being on her feet for a long time, which causes blood to collect and pool in her relaxed leg veins.
4. Swelling of the lower leg and ankle occurs because the back pressure from the distended veins causes fluid to leak out of capillary vessels into the tissues.
5. If she doesn't eat frequently, her blood sugar level falls.
6. Fatigue sets in.

Unfortunately for the woman and baby, this sequence of events creates the problems we described in chapter 2 for some of the physiological adaptations occurring in early pregnancy: not enough blood in the central circulation to maintain cardiac output and nutrient delivery at ideal levels (the underfill problem). As a result, both blood pressure and the rate of blood flow to the womb are reduced for protracted periods. This reduced blood flow, coupled with falling blood sugar, limits oxygen availability and decreases the nutrient supply to the baby, which slows growth of the baby and increases the irritability of the uterine muscle and the risk of premature labor (Clapp 1994b).

Once it was recognized that recreational exercise usually does not produce most of these effects—symptoms of severe fatigue, pooling of blood in the legs, or low blood pressure—investigators began to separately quantify physical stress on the job and physical stress from recreational exercise to determine if either is associated with premature labor or smaller than average babies. To date, all the studies indicate that recreational exercise has a different effect on pregnancy outcome. It does not increase the incidence of either smaller than average babies or premature labor; and it actually may decrease the incidence of both (Berkowitz et al. 1983; Klebanoff, Shiono, and Carey 1990; Luke et al. 1995; Rabkin et al. 1990).

Recreational exercise may actually decrease the chances of both premature labor and the birth of a very small baby.

Note that this finding fits nicely with ideas we have already discussed in chapter 2. For example, the physiological state created by the interaction between the functional adaptations to pregnancy and to exercise is protective against circulatory and metabolic stress in most situations. Now let's see if the same thing happens when women continue vigorous, sustained, weight-bearing exercise throughout mid- and late pregnancy.

Regular Exercise and Premature Birth

One question we asked when we began our studies was "Does continuing a regimen of sustained, weight-bearing exercise (running or aerobics as opposed to biking or swimming) throughout pregnancy increase the risk of premature labor?" We also asked "Do either sudden foot-strike shock or bouncing, ballistic motions cause the membranes that surround the baby to burst before they should?" To answer these questions, we established an accurate due date for each woman who enrolled in the study by obtaining an early pregnancy test, an accurate menstrual and sexual history, and an early ultrasound exam at seven and one-half to eight weeks after her last menstrual period. Then we monitored exercise performance throughout the pregnancy in the regularly exercising women who continued to perform sustained types of weight-bearing exercise at or above the basic fitness level throughout pregnancy (see next section). We compared the timing of their deliveries with those of a matched control group (women with active lifestyles who did not maintain a regular exercise regimen).

Exercise Characteristics

To remain in the exercise group, a woman had to meet two exercise performance criteria. First, she had to maintain her exercise regimen above 50 percent of her prepregnancy level. Second, her level of exercise also had to remain above that required to maintain basic fitness (three times a week, for 20 minutes at a moderately hard to hard level of perceived exertion). Thus, a woman who performed step aerobics five times a week before pregnancy but cut back to twice a week in mid- and late pregnancy was not included in the exercise group. The same was true for runners who dropped their weekly mileage by more than 50 percent even though they continued to run three times a week for 30 minutes at 65 percent of their maximum aerobic capacity.

More than 70 percent of the women in the exercise group, however, continued to meet the two exercise criteria for retention in the exercise group, and, in most cases, performance was much better than 50 percent of their prepregnancy level. Over the last three months, their average exercise intensity fell a little bit (from 66 to 59 percent of maximal aerobic capacity), but, in many cases, the time spent each week in exercise increased. As a result, the range in individual exercise performance or volume (the product of weekly intensity and duration) varied from a low of 50 to a high of 130 percent of prepregnancy levels with a group mean of 71 percent.

About half of the remaining women stopped regular sustained exercise completely by the 30th week and half cut back to much less than 50 percent of their prepregnancy levels. The main reason given was they felt that they no longer had enough time once they started preparing for the birth. The second reason was continuous pressure from people (mothers, husbands, friends, or doctors) who were concerned that the exercise might hurt the baby or initiate premature birth. The third reason was that they became concerned themselves. Physical discomfort was way down on the list, and injury did not play a role. As a matter of fact, of the over 250 exercising women we have studied, we have yet to encounter a woman who developed an exercise-associated injury that led to a cessation of exercise in late pregnancy.

We followed all the women and, therefore, have accurate information on the timing of delivery in three rather than two groups. More than 200 women continued a vigorous exercise regimen to within a week of delivery, and more than 80 women who exercised vigorously throughout early and midpregnancy cut back or stopped. The third group included about 250 physically active control women who rarely engaged in sustained exercise but occasionally played tennis, walked, gardened, and so on.

Study Results

When we examined the results, it was clear that the repetitive foot strike of running and the sudden motions of aerobics did not cause the membranes to burst (water to break) before the onset of labor at term. The chance that this would occur before the beginning of the 37th week was low and was the same in all three groups. This was also true at the end of pregnancy. Even after the mouth of the womb (cervix) had begun to dilate, women could continue to run or participate in aerobics without increasing the chance that the membranes surrounding the baby would burst before the onset of labor.

Continuing regular, vigorous exercise throughout pregnancy *does not* increase the incidence of either membrane rupture or preterm labor.

The gestational age when labor and delivery occurred is shown in figure 4.1 for the women who continued exercise and the physically active controls. It illustrates the percentage of women in each group who delivered each week, from the 32nd week through the end of the 42nd week, with term being the end of the 40th week.

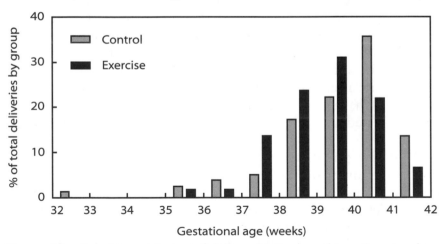

Figure 4.1 Exercise and timing of delivery. Notice two things: Exercise does not increase the number of premature births, and women who exercise deliver earlier at term.

Note that there is no suggestion that continuing regular exercise during pregnancy increases the incidence of delivering early enough to cause a problem related to prematurity for the baby (before the beginning of the 37th week). However, after the 37th week, we found a different story entirely. In each of the next three weeks, many more women who continued to exercise delivered. As a result, the number who delivered before their due date was much greater (72 percent) than in the control group (48 percent). Indeed, the control women didn't catch up with the exercising women until the second week after their due date, indicating that the timing of delivery at term was shifted to the left (earlier) for the entire exercise group. This means that a woman who continues regular, sustained exercise until the onset of labor usually delivers five to seven days earlier than a woman with an active lifestyle who does not exercise regularly. What an incentive to exercise! I'll bet if you ask any woman in the last month of her pregnancy, she'd give her right arm to deliver a few days early.

We also looked to see if there was a dose-response effect. Did the women who did the most exercise deliver earlier than those who did less? We couldn't detect any consistent relationship. Neither the absolute nor the relative amount of exercise made a difference, as long as they maintained their absolute exercise volume at or above 20 minutes of exercise, three times a week, at a moderately hard to hard level of perceived exertion.

Finally, the timing of delivery in the group of women who stopped exercising midpregnancy was no different from the controls. Thus, the timing of delivery at term is not altered if you exercise strenuously throughout early and midpregnancy, then stop. To be sure to get the benefit of delivering five to seven days earlier than you would if you didn't exercise, you must continue to exercise right until term. The amount of exercise it takes appears to be no more than that needed to maintain a basal level of fitness (three or more 20-minute sessions a week, at a moderately hard to hard level of perceived exertion). Cutting back to something below that level simply won't do the trick.

We have not been able to determine if there is either a type or an amount of exercise done in mid- and late pregnancy that will initiate labor ahead of schedule. It appears that even women who compete regularly before pregnancy and continue during pregnancy can maintain their exercise regimen at the same level throughout without increasing their risk. Although the numbers are smaller, it appears that they may even be able to exceed 100 percent of their prepregnancy exercise performance by 10 to 30 percent without increasing their risk of premature labor. But what about women who start an exercise program during pregnancy?

Starting a Fitness Program During Pregnancy

Unfortunately, no one has examined the effect of beginning a basic fitness program at about the time of conception or in early pregnancy. Over the last 15 years, however, there have been many studies examining the effect of beginning a fitness program in midpregnancy (Beckmann and Beckmann 1990; Collings, Curet, and Mullen 1983; Hall and Kaufmann 1987; Hatch et al. 1993; Kulpa, White, and Visscher 1987; Sibley et al. 1981; Wolfe et al. 1994). Participation has usually begun early in the fourth month and continued until term. The types of exercise in the studies have included swimming, stationary cycling, walking, and circuit training. In several, the women did enough exercise to provide evidence of improved fitness. Even when you combine the results (Lokey et al. 1991), however, the timing of the onset of labor has been no different from that of their more sedentary sisters.

Starting a regular exercise regimen during pregnancy *does not* increase the incidence of preterm labor.

These findings are different from our experience with women who continue exercising throughout their pregnancies. As many of these other exercise regimens varied from what the women in our studies did, we thought that the differences in results might be explained by differences in some aspect of the exercise regimens (type, frequency, intensity, or duration). To determine if this was the case, we recently began a series of prospective, randomized studies in which we control several of these factors and vary others. We allow only weight-bearing exercise (brisk walking, running, aerobics, stair climbing, and cross-country skiing), keep intensity at 55 percent of maximum capacity, and vary only the frequency (three to five times a week) and duration (20 to 60 minutes) of the exercise sessions.

The preliminary data from these studies indicate that starting to exercise in early pregnancy and continuing to term does not increase the chance of going into labor ahead of schedule. It does, however, increase the chance of delivering at term before the due date is reached. At this intensity, however, it appears that an increase in both the frequency and duration of weight-bearing exercise is necessary (40-minute sessions, four or more days each week) in women who have not been exercising regularly before pregnancy. Although these preliminary findings clearly support the idea that it is differences in the type of exercise prescribed or the frequency and duration of the exercise sessions that explain why others have not had similar results to ours, only time and studying a lot more subjects will tell for sure.

Effects of Regular Exercise on Fetal Growth

To establish the effect of regular exercise on the baby's growth, we did detailed measurements of all the babies born to the women in our study within 24 hours of birth. We measured the baby's weight, length, hat size (head circumference), pant size (abdominal circumference), and fatness (skinfold thicknesses) using a carefully standardized approach. We then compared these measurements in the three groups (exercise continued, control, exercise stopped). The results from comparing both exercise groups with the control groups are shown in figure 4.2. Table 4.1 compares all three groups.

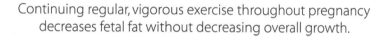

Continuing regular, vigorous exercise throughout pregnancy decreases fetal fat without decreasing overall growth.

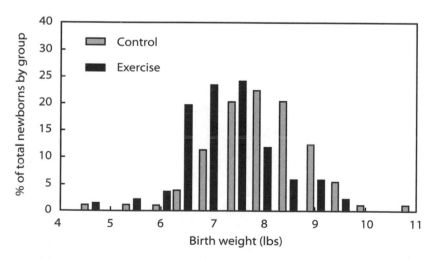

Figure 4.2   Exercise and birth weight. Notice two things: Women who exercise don't have low birth weight babies, but they do have more lighter babies and fewer big babies.

Figure 4.2 demonstrates that the distribution of birth weights of the babies delivered by women who continue to exercise shifted to the left. There were more babies in the exercise group who weighed less than seven and one-half pounds and fewer who weighed more. As a result of this shift, the average birth weight for the babies in the exercise group was 14 ounces lighter (7 pounds 2 ounces versus 8 pounds). In addition, the skinfold measurements indicated that they were thinner than the babies in the control group (11- versus 16-percent body fat). However, there was no increase in the incidence of *low birth weight* babies in the exercise group (less than 5 pounds 8 ounces, or 2,500 grams), and both length and head growth were unaffected. They grew their brains, organs, muscles, and bones at the same rate as the babies born to control women, but they didn't get as fat in the process. Thus, they have big heads and little bellies, and not much fat on their arms and legs. The best description I can think of to provide a visual image of what these babies look like compared to those born to the control women is that they are *lean*

Table 4.1

Effect of Regular Exercise During Pregnancy on Fetal Growth

	Exercise continued	Control	Exercise stopped
Weight (lb-oz)	7-2	8-0	8-8
Weight percentile	43	63	73
Length (in.)	20.24	20.24	20.35
Weight/length ratio	3.52	3.95	4.18
Head circumference (in.)	13.78	13.82	13.90
Abdominal circumference (in.)	12.44	13.46	14.00
Head/abdominal circumference ratio	1.11	1.03	.99
% body fat	10.70	15.90	18.70

Note: This table lists the mean values for the measurements obtained from the infants in the three groups. The higher the weight percentile, the bigger the baby relative to the other babies born at that gestational age. The higher the weight/length ratio, the bulkier the baby. The higher the head/abdominal circumference ratio, the leaner the baby.

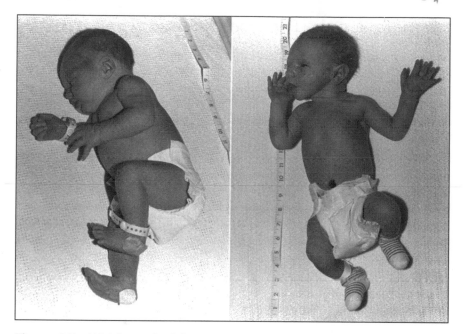

Figure 4.3   Which one had the exercising mom?

and mean. I've included a picture of two of them so you can see for yourself (see figure 4.3).

It also turned out that the amount of exercise a woman did in late pregnancy relative to what she did before pregnancy increased this lean and mean effect. For example, a woman who increased her weekly running mileage from 15 to 20 miles usually had a baby who weighed about a pound less than the baby born to a woman who cut her running from 35 to 25 miles a week in late pregnancy, even though the first woman's absolute weekly mileage was 25 percent lower than the second woman's.

Finally, if you add the difference in fat mass—about 8 ounces (percentage of birth weight that was fat in the control babies [20 ounces] minus that in the babies born to the women who exercised [12 ounces])—to the 3- to 4-ounce weight difference from being born five to seven days earlier (in late pregnancy the baby grows about 5 ounces a week), you can account for all the difference in birth weight. Thus, the only tissue whose growth has been reduced by the exercise is the baby's fat. So the next question (which we will answer later in chapter 7) is "Is it better to be bigger at birth if bigger is simply more fat?"

Stopping Regular Exercise Later in Pregnancy

As you can see from table 4.1, exercising vigorously early, then stopping in the latter part of pregnancy produces the biggest (eight pounds, eight ounces) and fattest (19 percent) babies of all. The reason for this appears to be that early exercise stimulates growth of the placenta (see "How Regular Exercise Affects Placental Growth" later in this chapter). Once the woman stops exercise, this provides the baby with a marked increase in available calories and nutrients, which stimulates continued growth. If you do the calculations, you will find that five and one-half ounces of this increase (about 70 percent) is due simply to an increase in fat mass.

Stopping exercise in late pregnancy tends to produce a larger baby who has more body fat.

Starting Regular Exercise During Pregnancy

The investigators mentioned earlier looked to see if the exercise programs they had prescribed influenced birth weight, and with one exception, they didn't find that it did. The one exception (Hatch et al. 1993) noted that starting a program of regular exercise during pregnancy increased birth weight unless the volume of exercise was very high. The preliminary data from our ongoing training studies suggest that starting exercise in the second month reduces birth weight and newborn fat mass, but only if the duration and frequency of the exercise are much higher (five days a week, for 40 minutes, at a moderately hard intensity) than that reported in these other training studies (three times a week for 15 to 20 minutes). In fact, our findings to date in women who are randomized to start and maintain a three-day-a-week, 20-minute regimen (Clapp, Tomaselli, Rizdon, et al. 1997) are quite similar to those reported earlier by Hatch and colleagues (1993).

How Regular Exercise Affects Placental Growth

We reasoned that if exercise affects growth of the baby it probably affects growth of the placenta as well. So we used a special ultrasound

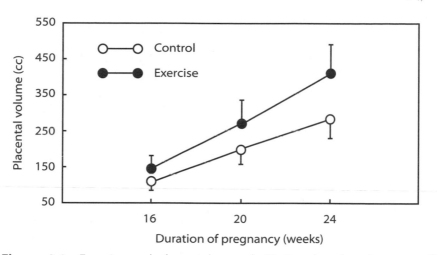

Figure 4.4   Exercise and placental growth. Notice that the placentae of women who exercise grow much faster than the placentae of women who don't.

technique to measure the growth rate of the placenta in a group of exercisers and controls during the middle of pregnancy (between the 16th and 24th week) when it is growing much faster than the baby, and we got the wonderful surprise illustrated in figure 4.4.

As you can see, this explained a lot. Exercise didn't slow down the growth of the placenta at all. Rather it increased it (Clapp and Rizk 1992), which ultimately improved its functional capacity in late pregnancy (Jackson et al. 1995). If exercise continued, the placenta grew almost a third faster in midpregnancy and had about 15 percent more vessels and surface area at term. This explains why a little bit of exercise throughout or exercising regularly then stopping in late pregnancy produces a big baby. It's another example of how the interaction between regular exercise and pregnancy produces an unanticipated protective effect that reduces fetal risk if complications develop late in pregnancy.

Summary

Now I'll review what we have observed about the interaction between exercise, premature labor, and the rate of growth of the baby and its placenta because it will be very important when I discuss designing a holistic exercise program. First, all the available evidence indicates that continuing or starting a regular exercise program does not increase a woman's chances of either rupturing her membranes or going into labor ahead of schedule, even if she exercises more during pregnancy than she did before she got pregnant. Furthermore, this appears to be true for many exercise modes, including running, many types of aerobics, cross-country skiing, stair stepping, swimming, biking, and circuit training. However, it appears that lots of weight-bearing exercise right until term does increase a woman's chances of delivering shortly before her due date by about 50 percent (a distinct plus if you happen to be the pregnant woman). Nonweight-bearing exercise does not alter the timing of labor, and the same is true in women who either continue weight-bearing exercise at a markedly reduced level or stop completely.

If a woman continues to exercise three times a week, for 20 minutes, at a moderately hard to hard level of perceived exertion throughout midpregnancy, that is enough to stimulate better than average placental growth and functional capacity. If a woman continues at that level throughout late pregnancy, that's enough to restrict excess fetal fat deposition without interfering with the growth of other fetal tissues. If, however, she cuts back or stops, all bets are off. Chances are she will have a much bigger and fatter baby. If she hasn't exercised before and starts to exercise during pregnancy for the first time, this amount of exercise will stimulate placental growth, but it takes almost twice as much exercise in late pregnancy to restrict excess fetal fat deposition. Next, we'll look at another area of concern, the impact of exercise during pregnancy on two postnatal events—lactation and growth in infancy.

CHAPTER 5

Exercise, Breast-Feeding, and Infant Growth

D uring sustained exercise, a woman loses water in sweat and expends between 300 and 600 kilocalories an hour. A woman breast-feeding a baby also expends an increasing number of calories to produce enough milk to satisfy a rapidly growing infant (usually exceeding 500 kilocalories by four months of age). Therefore, when sustained exercise and lactation are combined, several questions and concerns arise:

- Does exercise interfere with a woman's ability to produce enough milk to satisfy her infant's needs?
- Does it change the quality of the milk she produces by either altering its protein, fat, and carbohydrate content or adding fixed acids that might alter taste?
- If so, does regular exercise during lactation slow infant growth?

What follows provides the best answers currently available. It is a detailed review of the results from several recent studies that specifically explored the issues of exercise, milk production, and infant growth.

How Exercise Affects Milk Production

The concern that regular exercise during lactation alters the quality and quantity of the breast milk had its origins in the dairy science literature, which indicated that even modest increases in physical activity decreased milk production in cows (Lamb, Anderson, and Walters 1979). This was reinforced in the early 1990s by the finding that high-intensity exercise increased the levels of lactic acid in human milk to a level which altered its taste and decreased infant suckling (Wallace, Inbar, and Ernsthausen 1992).

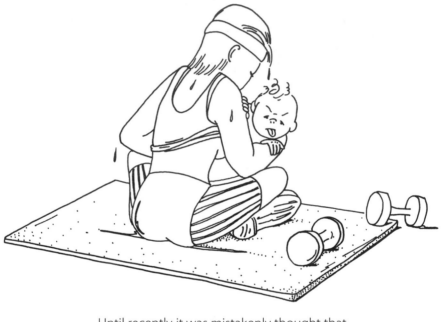

Until recently, it was mistakenly thought that exercise adversely affected milk taste.

Unfortunately, these findings were interpreted too broadly (guilt by association again), which reinforced the recommendation that women breast-feeding their babies should curtail their exercise for a protracted time after the birth. However, the findings also stimulated multiple studies to determine exactly what effect a regular program of exercise had on milk production, nursing behavior, and infant growth. The best of these was a series of detailed studies by a group of nutritionists in California. They demonstrated that frequent, sustained, moderate- to high-intensity running during lactation did not impair the quantity or quality of human breast milk (Dewey et al. 1994; Dewey and McCrory 1994; Lovelady, Lonnerdal, and Dewey 1990). Unfortunately, they did not measure lactic acid levels in the milk to determine if they were elevated by the exercise regimen. (High levels of lactic acid in breast milk can give it a sour taste.) Still, the results indicated that the exercise regimen did not noticeably affect infant nursing behavior (Dewey and Lovelady 1993) suggesting that the lactic acid content of breast milk was not great enough to cause a sour or unpleasant taste.

The experience of my laboratory is similar. Our subjects do not report any difficulty with infant receptivity that they associate with their exercise patterns. This finding appears to hold true for most but not all competitive women who continue to train at high levels (perceived exertion hard to very hard, for more than 60 minutes on a regular basis). It is also true for the average women who participate in our studies (perceived exertion moderate to hard, for 20 to 50 minutes three to seven times a week). To be sure that this is the case, we have begun a series of prospective studies to examine the lactic acid issue in breast milk under conditions of everyday life. To date, our findings agree with those published by Quinn and Carey (1997). Namely, unless exercise intensity is very high (above the aerobic threshold), there is little change in lactate levels in either maternal blood or breast milk.

Why are there such differences in the findings in this area? Everybody's findings are clear-cut. It appears that the reason for the discrepancies has to do with differences in the way each study approached the question. Remember, when investigators design an experiment, they usually do it in a way that provides a clear answer to their question. However, often we cannot apply that answer broadly because the experiment was limited to specific circumstances.

Regular, vigorous, aerobic exercise at moderate to
high intensity *does not* alter the quality
or quantity of breast milk in women.
However, extremely intense anaerobic exercise
(interval workouts) occasionally alters the taste of breast milk.

For instance, in the 1979 dairy study, Lamb and colleagues used forced exercise in a species of sedentary animals whose peak level of milk production is easily decreased by a variety of environmental factors. Therefore, the probability was high that they would demonstrate an effect, but it was unlikely that it would apply to the human condition. Wallace and colleagues (1992) used short periods of intense exercise that clearly exceeded the women's anaerobic thresholds. As blood lactate levels rise rapidly once the anaerobic threshold is reached, the likelihood was high that lactic acid levels in the breast milk would increase much more than they would with a representative exercise session, causing the milk to taste sour.

In contrast, the three studies by Dewey's group (1991, 1993, 1994) focused on a more practical problem—the effects of exercise and lactation on postpartum weight loss. Can a woman combine a rigorous exercise regimen with lactation to speed maternal weight loss without impairing the quantity and quality of milk production or infant growth? To answer it, they used a representative exercise stimulus—frequent, prolonged exercise sessions at intensities below the anaerobic threshold.

Likewise, our subjects exercised at their usual intensities for their usual time, and, when tested in a laboratory setting, their intensities were below their anaerobic threshold. Thus our preliminary findings, those of Quinn and Carey (1997), and the multiple studies by Dewey's group (1991; 1993; 1994) are more representative of what happens in everyday life. As such, they probably provide a more valid reference for counseling women who wish to continue their exercise regimen during lactation. The information from Wallace and colleagues probably applies only to women who plan frequent, high-intensity interval training. Indeed, more recent results from her laboratory indicate that only minor increases in lactic acid content occur after usual workouts, and these small changes do not noticeably affect infant suckling behavior (Wallace, Inbar, and Ernsthausen 1994). So, most of the time the relationship between the mother and suckling infant is what you see in figure 5.1, exercise or not.

As a whole, this information supports the view that healthy breast-feeding women may continue to exercise if they wish. On the one hand, most women can assume a high level of exercise performance or training while breast-feeding without interfering with either the quantity or quality of breast milk. Clearly they can do enough to regain, maintain, or improve their fitness level long before they stop breast-feeding. On the other hand, there apparently are a few women whose infants don't nurse well after a sustained, moderate-intensity exercise session. However, this probably is due to other as yet undefined factors (infant hunger, maternal odor, sweat, degree of relaxation, etc.) rather than a

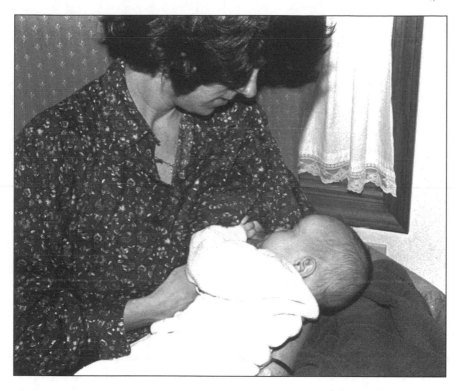

Figure 5.1 Usual breast-feeding experience after exercise.

high level of lactic acid in the breast milk. Likewise, frequent interval training at an intensity that exceeds a woman's anaerobic threshold may alter taste and decrease infant receptivity due to an increase in lactic acid levels in the milk. Short of that it appears that the exercise threshold required to decrease the quality and quantity of milk is high, variable among individuals, and remains to be established.

Maternal Weight Loss While Breast-Feeding

There are two other important questions that sometimes come up about exercise and milk production.

- Is it all right to exercise regularly, breast-feed, and diet to lose weight at the same time?

- Will the combination of caloric restriction and exercise change the quantity or quality of breast milk?

These questions come up because women, especially athletic women, want to get back to their prepregnant weight rapidly and often are discouraged by their rate of weight loss a month or two after the birth. The concern about answering the first question with a direct *yes* originates from studies that examined the effect of changes in maternal nutrition during lactation in baboons. These studies indicate that both mild and moderate caloric restriction (80 and 60 percent of maintenance caloric requirements) decrease milk production and infant growth, even though baboon mothers reduce their activity when their calories are restricted (Roberts, Cole, and Coward 1985).

A woman can breast-feed, exercise, and diet
at the same time, but she should limit
caloric restriction and her rate of weight loss.

These provocative findings initiated a study in healthy, breast-feeding, but nonexercising women in which maternal caloric intake was acutely restricted an average of 38 percent for one week (Strode, Dewey, and Lonnerdal 1986). The caloric restriction increased maternal weight loss without altering milk quantity or quality. When the data were examined carefully, however, this was only true for women who continued to eat more than 1,500 kilocalories a day. Women who reduced their intakes below 1,500 kilocalories a day (more than a 30-percent reduction in caloric intake) did experience a decrease in milk production, and infant weight gain decreased as well. These findings are similar to the early baboon studies.

The definitive study has not been done yet (dieting and exercising while breast-feeding). However, the findings of these two studies, combined with information on lactation in marginally nourished women in third-world countries, suggest that there must be a reasonable balance between a lactating woman's energy intake and energy expenditure. If her caloric intake falls well below her caloric expenditure, then it will decrease milk production and probably infant weight gain as well. The threshold for this effect is when calories in are about 20 to 25 percent below calories out, but, in practice, the value will undoubtedly vary from woman to woman, culture to culture, and may also be influenced by breast-feeding practices (frequency, duration, and so on).

So, we don't have all the answers about whether it's OK for a woman to exercise and diet while she is breast-feeding. However, these and other experiments that we discuss in the next chapter suggest that there is a practical, safe answer to the question. That answer is, as long as the baby doesn't mind (i.e., isn't a cranky, unhappy baby who always wants to suckle) and infant weight gain is normal, it's OK to exercise, diet, and breast-feed as long as you don't lose weight faster than three-quarters of a pound to a pound a week. There is one additional caveat: when babies enter a growth spurt their caloric needs increase which leads to an increase in suckling frequency that stimulates the breast to produce the extra milk required; until the breasts' production of milk increases to meet these demands many babies get cranky. So the dieting, nursing mother must learn to differentiate between the effects of her excessive caloric restriction and the effects of a normal growth spurt on her infant's behavior. The best clue is that the former produces continuous discontent and poor weight gain in the infant while the effect of the latter is limited and sporadic.

When a sensible program of caloric restriction is combined with regular exercise and breast-feeding the rate of postpartum weight loss is roughly three times faster than usual when breast-feeding, exercising women eat to appetite. It represents an energy deficit of about 425 kilocalories a day, which is between 15 and 20 percent of anticipated energy requirements for most exercising, lactating women. Most women who elect to follow this type of regimen should do so with the guidance of a nutritionist to be sure that the quality of their caloric intake remains adequate.

Breast-Feeding and Infant Growth

Another question to answer is whether breast-feeding alters the pattern or the rate of infant growth. With the resurgence of breast-feeding in the 1980s, pediatricians noted that many exclusively breast-fed infants had a reduced caloric intake and did not grow as rapidly as formula-fed infants after two to three months of age (Butte et al. 1984). This led to a detailed series of studies, which examined energy intake, growth, and development of breast-fed infants through the first two years of life (Dewey et al. 1991, 1992, 1993, 1995, 1996).

These studies confirmed that both the caloric intake and weight gain of breast-fed infants were less than those of formula-fed infants. However, there was no evidence that the breast-fed infants were either underfed or hungry. Rather, they appeared satisfied with their caloric intake and actually stopped feeding even though milk remained in the breast.

Breast-fed infants are naturally leaner than bottle-fed infants.

Interestingly enough, their growth pattern was similar to the one we have observed at birth in the babies born to women who exercise. Their growth in length and head circumference was the same as formula-fed infants, protein supplementation did not increase their growth rates, they were healthy, and they reached their developmental milestones on schedule. It turned out that, apart from weight gain, the only difference was that they didn't deposit as much fat! Thus, the pattern of weight gain is different for infants who are breast-fed because they are leaner than formula-fed babies. So when we examine the effects of exercise on infant growth, we must compare breast-fed infants to breast-fed infants. A word of caution: if a question arises about the adequacy of growth in a breast-fed infant, check that the chart being used was developed for breast-fed babies. Out of habit, many health professionals still use charts based on the growth rates of formula-fed babies.

Effects of Exercise During Lactation on Infant Growth

Now we can ask "Does regular, sustained exercise during lactation alone or during pregnancy and lactation alter the pattern of infant growth in exclusively breast-fed infants?" Unfortunately, we can't effectively study exercise and pregnancy without lactation as, in our 15-year experience, less than two percent of women who exercise during pregnancy feed formula to their offspring.

Regular exercise during lactation *does not* slow infant growth.

The studies from Dewey's group looked at this question carefully and concluded that the growth of breast-fed infants was not impaired in any way by a taxing exercise program during lactation (Dewey et al. 1994; Lovelady, Lonnerdal, and Dewey 1990). However, they only observed and measured a limited number of babies over a 12-week period. Our ongoing study has produced similar findings. Although not as well controlled, it extends over a longer time and involves a larger number of infants whose mothers exercised and breast-fed them (Clapp 1996a, 1996b; Clapp, Simonian, et al. 1995). To date we have gathered preliminary data in over 50 matched pairs at one year of age to determine if exercise during pregnancy and lactation alters the pattern of infant growth. The data indicate that continuing a regular program of exercise throughout pregnancy and lactation does not alter weight, length, head circumference, or fat mass at one year of age, and, at age five, the only difference is that the exercise offspring are leaner.

These findings reinforce the view that healthy, breast-feeding women can continue to exercise without compromising the growth and development of their offspring. Again, they indicate that most healthy women can begin or continue an exercise regimen rigorous enough to regain, maintain, or improve their fitness level during lactation without interfering with infant growth. Furthermore, they suggest that, if unidentified problems with infant receptivity do occur after exercise (especially high-intensity training such as interval training), they are not of sufficient magnitude to create a demonstrable difference in infant growth. Finally, in the absence of severe maternal caloric restriction, the exercise threshold required to alter the growth of a breast-fed infant must be high and remains to be established.

The impact of exercise on lactation and infant growth is the last of the major concerns about maternal exercise that I specifically discuss. I mention others briefly in the next two chapters where we turn our attention to the benefits of regular, sustained exercise during pregnancy and lactation for the mother and baby.

Summary

Although initially an area of legitimate concern, work over the last decade supports the view that beginning or continuing a regular exercise regimen during lactation does not have adverse effects on milk production or infant growth if the woman is healthy and not restricting her caloric intake unduly. This view is supported by a large volume of experimental findings gathered about breast-feeding women who did many forms of exercise, at moderate or high intensities, for both short and long periods, as frequently as six times a week.

There are only two exceptions and one *maybe* identified to date. First, intense interval training may alter the taste and infant acceptance of breast milk right after a training session. Second, infant acceptability of breast milk can decrease occasionally in a woman after a moderate-intensity workout for reasons that are unclear at present. The *maybe* involves the question of whether it is wise for an exercising, breast-feeding woman to diet. Although the final answer is not in yet, it appears that a moderate reduction in caloric intake can be well tolerated by the woman and not impair the function of her breasts or the growth of her baby. Right now, outside of a change in the baby's response, the best guide to how much of a reduction in calories is OK is for the woman to keep her rate of weight loss under one pound a week.

CHAPTER 6

Maternal Benefits of Regular Exercise

In looking at the question of maternal benefits, it is important to recognize that the word exercise means different things to different people. From what we've said already, it's clear that many things people call exercise do not have negative effects on the course and outcome of pregnancy. However, many of these regimens do not provide enough exercise stimulus to benefit the pregnancy either.

This chapter attempts to establish the *threshold* level of exercise—the least amount of exercise a woman must do to obtain the maternal benefits. Then I discuss whether the amount of exercise she does above that threshold level increases the benefit she obtains and determine if there is a so-called dose-response effect. I also identify the exercise variables (type, frequency, intensity, and duration) that appear to be most important in achieving each of several benefits.

I examine a fairly wide range of benefits, including some objective ones like fitness, weight gain, and length of labor. In addition, I discuss some that are difficult to quantify objectively, such as attitudes, immune function, and feelings of well-being. I also look for beneficial effects in three groups of women (those who continue regular exercise throughout pregnancy, those who continue then stop, and those who start for the first time during pregnancy) to determine if the timing of the exercise in pregnancy makes a difference.

Let's begin with the effects of exercise that we can easily and objectively measure. These include

- maternal weight gain and fat accumulation,
- maternal discomfort and injury,
- the course and outcome of labor,
- pregnancy complications, and
- maternal physical fitness.

Reduced Maternal Weight Gain and Fat Accumulation

When we began these studies, we asked whether regular exercise restricts weight gain during pregnancy and, if so, when and what tissues are affected. Our initial observations indicated that weight gain averaged about 3.6 kilograms (8 pounds) less in women who continued to exercise throughout pregnancy (Clapp and Capeless 1990). This led to several detailed studies in which we made serial measurements of weight gain and five site skinfold thicknesses before, during, and after pregnancy (Clapp and Little 1995; Little, Clapp, and Ridzon 1994, 1995).

Continuing Regular Exercise Throughout Pregnancy

The effect of continuing regular exercise throughout pregnancy on weight gain and fat deposition is illustrated in figures 6.1 and 6.2.

As you can see, we found that continuing exercise throughout pregnancy had a marked influence on weight gain, fat deposition, and fat retention. Furthermore, the effect was much more pronounced in the second half of pregnancy (after the 20th week). Overall weight gain was reduced by a little more than three kilograms, or seven pounds (see figure 6.1), and skinfolds by 15 millimeters. This difference in the change in skinfold thicknesses indicated that body fat mass increased approximately three percent less in the women who continued regular weight-bearing exercise (see figure 6.2), and the more exercise these women did in late pregnancy, the greater the effect on both weight gain and fat retention. Note (in figures 6.1 and 6.2) that the between-group differences in weight and skinfolds were small until the second half of pregnancy, when more than 75 percent of the differences developed. The end result is that the women who continue to exercise maintain a lean appearance throughout pregnancy, and, as shown in figure 6.3, if you can't see their abdomens, they don't look pregnant! Believe

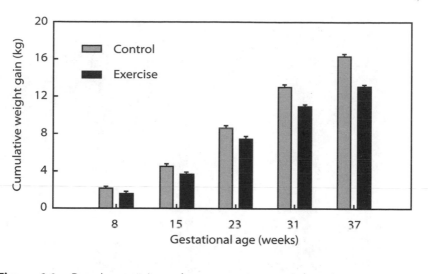

Figure 6.1   Regular exercise reduces pregnancy weight gain.

me, this helps many women with their body image during pregnancy. It does not mean, however, that these women are either underfed or malnourished. The average increases in weight (13 kilograms, or 29 pounds) and skinfold thicknesses (10 millimeters) in these women are well within the normal range for pregnancy.

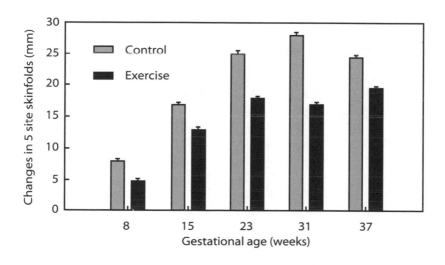

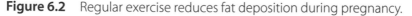

Figure 6.2   Regular exercise reduces fat deposition during pregnancy.

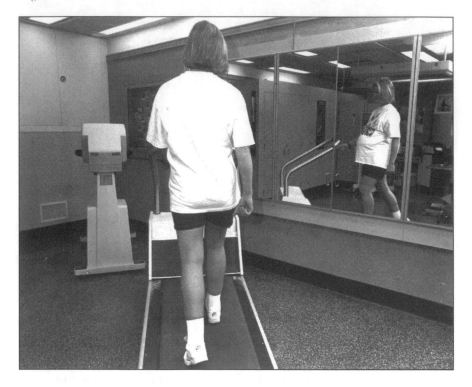

Figure 6.3   Exercise and physical appearance late in pregnancy, back versus front.

Postpartum Exercise

After these findings, we were astonished to learn that continuing regular exercise after the birth did not have the same effect on the postpartum loss of either weight or fat. As a matter of fact, the exercise effect was minimal! The differences in weight loss were less than two pounds over a three-month interval, and there was no difference in fat loss at all (figure 6.4). We just didn't understand how this could be. At first we thought that we must have made a mistake, but even after we had studied more women, the results were the same. Also, Dewey's group in California found exactly the same pattern (Dewey et al. 1994; Lovelady, Lonnerdal, and Dewey 1990). Although their breast-feeding women maintained a vigorous weight-bearing exercise regimen (400 or more kilocalories a day), the women's rate of weight and fat loss was identical to that of the women who did not exercise.

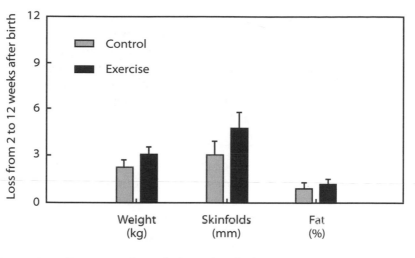

Figure 6.4   Exercise and weight loss after the birth.

Continuing regular exercise during pregnancy limits weight
gain and fat deposition in women, but exercise alone will not
increase the rate of weight loss after birth.

Fortunately, the researchers assessed one additional factor that affects weight stability, and that information explains why this vigorous
exercise regimen had little or no effect on the rate of weight loss. They
did careful measurements of caloric intake (what went in) as well as
caloric expenditure (what went out) and found that breast-feeding
women who exercise increase their daily food intake to cover their own
energy needs (daily life plus exercise) and those of their babies (milk
production). This explained the riddle. It was so simple we should have
thought of it! If you increase caloric intake to match caloric demand or
output, then weight doesn't change.

Beginning Regular Exercise During Pregnancy

Now comes the critical question that many women ask once they are
pregnant: If I start exercising now, will I cut down my weight gain for
the rest of pregnancy? Unfortunately, few studies have looked criti-
cally at the effect of beginning an exercise program during pregnancy

on weight gain, and those that have were unable to document an effect (Collings, Curet, and Mullen 1983). However, most of these programs started in midpregnancy with a limited amount of exercise, and, in many instances, the exercise was nonweight-bearing. This suggested to us that the amount of exercise necessary to influence weight gain may have been below the threshold level in these studies.

Starting regular, moderate-intensity exercise
during pregnancy will limit weight gain
and fat deposition but only if a woman exercises
more than three hours a week.

To check this possibility, we have kept exercise type (weight-bearing) and intensity (55 percent of maximum capacity) constant in our training programs, only varying frequency and duration. Our findings (Clapp, Tomaselli, et al. 1996) indicate that the exercise threshold necessary to achieve a weight gain and fat deposition reduction for someone starting exercise at the beginning of the third month is somewhere between 20 minutes, three to five times a week, and 40 minutes, five times a week. At the lower level, the changes are similar to those in the physically active control women (see figures 6.1 and 6.2). At the upper level, the changes are similar to those in women who continue their preconceptional exercise regimen throughout pregnancy.

Thus, the amount of exercise required to modify weight gain and fat retention during pregnancy is much greater for women who start an exercise program during pregnancy, compared to the exercise threshold for women who are already fit and continue to exercise during pregnancy.

Right now it is unclear why this is the case. One likely explanation is that a woman must expend a certain percentage of her daily caloric intake in exercise to modify weight gain and fat retention. Because the absolute caloric expenditure of a previously untrained woman exercising at 55 percent of her maximal capacity is less than that of a fit one exercising at the same intensity, the untrained woman must exercise a lot longer than the fit woman to expend the same number of calories. In any case, it appears that the answer to the question (does regular weight-bearing exercise during pregnancy limit weight gain?) can be either "yes" or "no," depending on prior training and the type, frequency, and duration of the exercise regimen.

Stopping Exercise in Midpregnancy

What about women who stop or cut way back on their exercise during pregnancy? You guessed it! They quickly catch up to the physically active, nonexercising controls, then pass them in late pregnancy. As a result, their overall weight gain is a bit more (about five pounds), and they accumulate a bit more fat (one to two percent) than the control women. As yet we have not determined why women who stop exercise gain more weight. The most likely explanation, however, is that they stop exercising (decrease caloric usage) without changing their caloric intake.

Less Maternal Discomfort and Injury

The effect of beginning or continuing a regular exercise program during pregnancy on the incidence of maternal discomfort due to either the exercise or the pregnancy is an unexplored area. The same is true for maternal injury. Nonetheless, the lack of reports of injury, soreness, and so on suggest to us that the incidence of exercise-associated discomforts and injuries probably do not increase during pregnancy (Sherer and Schenker 1989). In addition, when we reviewed the data obtained from the initial 100 women, we identified only one injury (a joint dislocation during a cross-country ski race in early pregnancy). The incidence of documented low-back, leg, or pelvic discomfort was less than 10 percent in the exercisers and greater than 40 percent in the controls. To be sure that both of these impressions are correct, we have kept track of the incidence of injury and discomfort in women who begin exercise during pregnancy, those who continue, and the physically active control women. To date, the findings (which follow) confirm our earlier impressions.

Unfortunately, we really don't understand what specific aspect of these women's exercise routines contributes to the improvement in well-being. To date we have not put specific emphasis on stretching, flexibility, or strength. The only common denominator is that the exercise sessions are regular, weight-bearing, and sustained.

Continuing Exercise Throughout Pregnancy

What about women who simply continue their usual exercise regimen throughout pregnancy? If anything, they decrease their risk of injury (Clapp 1994a). To date the exercise-associated injury rate is lower— about one percent, which is less than half that seen in the control group with the routine activities of everyday life. The three additional exercise-associated injuries seen to date include reactivation of an old ankle injury, precipitated by running on uneven terrain late in pregnancy; a metatarsal stress fracture in a high-mileage runner; and a bruise secondary to a fall while in-line skating. None of these injuries, however, were severe enough to necessitate a cessation of exercise in mid- to late pregnancy.

To date, there have been eight injuries in the controls. Three have been precipitated by a fall, two acute low-back syndromes were related to changes in posture associated with removing objects from car trunks, and three miscellaneous sprains (two ankles, one knee) had no clear etiology. In contrast to the exercisers, some of the injuries in these women (especially the low-back syndromes) resulted in physical limitations for extended periods of time.

Starting or continuing regular exercise during pregnancy and the postpartum period decreases physical discomforts, hastens recovery, and *does not* increase the risk of exercise-related injury.

Women who continue to exercise throughout pregnancy also experience fewer pregnancy discomforts and symptomatology. The incidence of specific physical complaints ranges between 10 and 40 percent of that seen in the physically active controls, which agrees with the only other report in this area (Wallace et al. 1986). However, about 20 percent of the women who continue to either run or do high-impact aerobics mention that they often experience lower abdominal discomfort or pelvic pressure during their exercise sessions in late pregnancy. Women can often relieve this by wearing maternity lower abdominal support belts that are commercially available (the use of one of these belts is illustrated in chapter 10). This suggests that the origin of the discomfort and pressure is excessive uterine mobility.

Postpartum Exercise

What about women who stop exercising for a few days before delivery, then start again shortly after the baby is born and continue throughout lactation? Are they uncomfortable? Do they hemorrhage, develop abdominal hernias, dropped bladders, and sagging wombs?

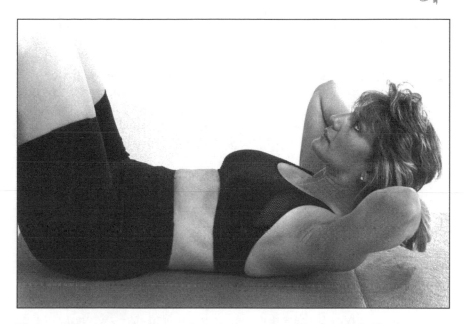

Figure 6.5 Abdominal crunches three weeks after the birth. She has great muscle tone, and it's her third baby.

Most women we have studied who exercised during pregnancy start again within two weeks of delivery. We check to see how they are doing six weeks, three months, six months, and a year after the birth. The photo in figure 6.5 was taken three weeks after delivery and illustrates how well these women feel physically and how fit they are. When compared to the physically active controls, the exercising women uniformly report a more rapid physical and emotional recovery (about twice as fast). The incidence of significant postpartum depression is also low. Perhaps this is because the time spent exercising is *personal* or *alone* time for the women and gives them a regular break from the 24-hour, seven-day-a-week commitment that comes with a new baby. As a result they don't appear to feel as overwhelmed and readily master the coping skills a new baby requires.

In addition, these women experience little in the way of discomfort during exercise. Women who start within a week of delivery, however, usually note a definite increase in vaginal bleeding during and immediately after exercise, but it has not been excessive and is usually gone within a week. Likewise, some runners note transitory feelings of instability at the hips, but, with one exception in our studies (reactivation of a chronic sacroiliac joint problem), pain has not been a problem.

Although the range of hyperextension at several joints is still increased for a time after the birth (Schauberger et al. 1996), there is nothing to suggest that this has functional significance or persists long term. A variety of floor exercises including different types of abdominal crunches rapidly improve abdominal muscle tone and have not caused hernias near or below the belly button. Indeed, as illustrated in figure 6.5, the abdominal wall musculature postpartum is often equal to or better than that observed prepregnancy.

Resuming regular exercise shortly after delivery has multiple benefits and does not cause long-term problems.

Some women who exercise postpartum experience some loss of urine during exercise in the first six weeks after the birth, but this problem clears up rapidly and does not reappear. Indeed, the frequency of its occurrence during everyday activity, coughing, or laughing is much less in exercisers than in the controls. Likewise, internal exams of the exercisers at six weeks have not shown evidence of poor vaginal or uterine support. Moreover, we have been unable to document a relationship between early resumption of exercise and infection, poor healing, or sexual malfunction. Finally, to be sure of the long-term maternal effects of exercise during pregnancy and after the birth, we have begun a detailed evaluation of the relationship among continuing regular exercise during and after pregnancy and potential problems with breastfeeding, weight, abdominal tone, bladder control, and sexual function. We've studied a matched group of these women one to two years after the birth. A preliminary analysis of these data indicates the following:

- 95 percent of the women who exercised regularly prior to pregnancy return to regular jogging, aerobics, or stair climbing after the birth.
- 40 percent return to regular exercise in the first two weeks after the birth at a light to moderately hard level of perceived exertion (average perceived level of exertion for these women prior to pregnancy was hard).
- Six months after the birth, they were all back to their normal level of perceived exertion, but only 66 percent felt that they had reached their prepregnancy fitness level.

- At six months, 55 percent had returned to their prepregnant weight and percent body fat; 75 percent at one year.
- At one year, the average abdominal tone rating was 15 percent lower than prior to pregnancy.
- Exercise did not cause either a loss of pelvic support or sexual dysfunction.
- 75 percent experienced no exercise-related problems.
- Two women reported an exercise-related problem with either their breasts or breast-feeding.
- Two experienced urinary incontinence during exercise.
- Five had musculoskeletal complaints.

When these data were compared with those collected from the physically active controls we found the following:

- Only 30 percent of controls (versus 65 percent of exercisers) stated that they had regained their prepregnancy fitness level.
- At one year, the average weight retention in the controls was three times greater and fat retention twice that seen in the exercisers.
- At one year, using a rating scale, the control women had an average abdominal tone rating that had decreased to 48 percent of prepregnancy levels (versus 85 percent in the exercisers).
- No difference was evident in the incidence of breast-feeding problems.
- No difference in the incidence or degree of urinary incontinence after the birth was evident, but the duration of nonexercise-induced incontinence (lifting, coughing, and so on) was much shorter in the exercisers (less than one month) than in the controls (three months to a year).
- No difference was found in various indexes of sexual function.

Thus, in most instances, women who continue exercise throughout pregnancy and begin again shortly after the birth do not experience pain; instead, they reap multiple emotional and physical benefits without compromising breast, bladder, or sexual function.

Beginning Regular Exercise During Pregnancy

Most women who begin a training program develop some initial muscle soreness that disappears within the first week or two. However, despite our studies' exclusive use of weight-bearing exercise, we have not seen a single injury in the beginning exerciser. Moreover, they repeatedly comment about how comfortable they are and how well they feel. Even late in pregnancy, back or hip discomfort has been rare and has not restricted activity. Most beginners do note, however, increasing pelvic pressure or an occasional stitch in the side during exercise in late pregnancy (after 32 weeks). In most instances, they can relieve this with lower abdominal support using either a wide Ace bandage wrap or a maternity abdominal support belt. Again, the beginning exercisers have fewer physical complaints related to the pregnancy than the physically active controls. This appears to be true for all exercising groups, even those who are exercising at the minimal level. Exercise or not, however, difficulty sleeping in late pregnancy is a universal problem.

Stopping Exercise in Midpregnancy

What about women who continue exercising early in the pregnancy then stop midpregnancy? Once they stop, they experience a gradual but distinct increase in the usual pregnancy-related physical symptomatology. Fatigue, leg aches, and low-back pain often appear, but they never reach the frequency or the intensity seen in the physically active control women.

Labor and Delivery Benefits

The reports on this topic are mixed. Most studies report that beginning exercise during pregnancy has no effect on the course and outcome of labor (Hatch et al. 1993; Lokey et al. 1991). Two anecdotal reports indicate that labor is probably prolonged in Olympic athletes (Erdelyi 1962; Zaharieva 1972), and two others found that regular exercise shortens it (Beckmann and Beckmann 1990; Wong and McKenzie 1987). The variance in these results was precisely what we had seen earlier when we looked at the issue of exercise and weight gain. Again, this variance led us to conclude that exercise probably does have an effect, but the effect had been obscured by differences in the exercise regimens, small sample sizes, and the errors inherent in the way the data were collected (retrospectively reviewing patient records after the delivery, rather than observing and recording all aspects of the course of labor as they happened).

Therefore, when we began our studies, we planned our approach to this question carefully. We set up objective criteria for progress in labor as well as the other outcome variables and arranged for a member of the study team to be present throughout labor and delivery to track exactly what happened when.

Continuing Exercise Throughout Pregnancy

We began by comparing the course and outcome of labor in the women who continued regular exercise throughout pregnancy with that of the physically active controls. As anticipated, we found that continuing weight-bearing exercise at the intensity, duration, and frequency detailed earlier had multiple positive effects on the labor and delivery.

Women who continue regular weight-bearing exercise throughout pregnancy tend to have easier, shorter, and less complicated labors.

First, as shown in table 6.1, there was a marked decrease in the need for all types of medical intervention for the exercising women. This included the following:

- A 35-percent decrease in the need for pain relief
- A 75-percent decrease in the incidence of maternal exhaustion
- A 50-percent decrease in the need to artificially rupture the membranes

Table 6.1

Effect of Exercise on the Course of Labor

	Exercise continued	Control	Exercise stopped
Pain relief	51	78	81
Labor stimulation	29	58	53
Fetal intervention	13	26	12
Forceps delivery	5	18	20
Cesarean section	9	29	26
Spontaneous delivery	86	53	54

Note: Data presented as the percentage of women in each group who required or experienced each intervention or nonintervention.

- A 50-percent decrease in the need to either induce or stimulate labor with pitocin
- A 50-percent decrease in the need to intervene because of abnormalities in the fetal heart rate
- A 55-percent decrease in the need for episiotomy (a cut between the vagina and rectum to give the baby more room to deliver)
- A 75-percent decrease in the need for operative intervention (either forceps delivery or cesarean section)

As a result, the women who continued to exercise had a striking increase (more than 30 percent) in the incidence of uncomplicated, spontaneous delivery, and, as shown in figure 6.6, the duration of active labor was much shorter. Again, the difference was large. Among the women with vaginal births, the length of labor was more than a third shorter in the women who continued to exercise than it was in the controls. More than 65 percent of the exercising women delivered in less than four hours, versus 31 percent in the controls. At the other extreme, active labor lasted between 10 and 14 hours in about 15 percent of the control women, and all the exercising women delivered in less than 10 hours. We saw similar between-group differences in duration in each of the two phases of active labor in women having their first or second delivery. On average, the breathing and relaxing phase was 90 to 100 minutes longer, and the pushing or expulsive phase was 30 to 40 minutes longer for the physically active controls. The average times were longer with first deliveries and shorter with second deliveries in both the exercise and control groups.

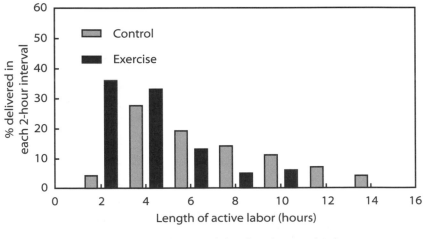

Figure 6.6   Regular exercise shortens labor by about a third.

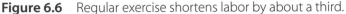

Beginning Regular Exercise During Pregnancy

Now the important public health question—will beginning an exercise program during pregnancy decrease the need for medical intervention and increase the rate of uncomplicated spontaneous delivery at term? I think so, but I can't answer that question with certainty right now. Most studies by other investigators report that exercise has no effect on the need for medical intervention or the incidence of uncomplicated, spontaneous delivery at term. Only a few studies report minimal benefit. These findings are different from our experiences with women who continue exercise, which again suggest that benefits in this area may relate to the type, frequency, duration, and intensity of the exercise. To date, the preliminary data from our training study support this interpretation, but not enough women in our training study have delivered to be sure that this is the case. However, both these preliminary data and the findings discussed earlier about women who continue to exercise, indicate that, to obtain this benefit, it is important to keep exercising regularly until near the onset of labor.

Stopping Exercise in Midpregnancy

What about the women who stopped regular exercise in midpregnancy? As shown in table 6.1, they did not experience during labor any benefits of regular exercise. Indeed, they were no different from the controls.

Effects on Potential Pregnancy Complications

Unfortunately, most studies have not examined the relationship between regular exercise and medical complications during pregnancy, so there is little information available. What is available suggests that there is little or no effect of exercise on complications. That is probably because the incidence of these complications is low, and, as yet, the number of women studied has not been large enough to detect a difference (Lokey et al. 1991).

Continuing Exercise Throughout Pregnancy

Our laboratory has looked at the incidence of several complications in the women we have studied, and the rates are either unaffected or reduced somewhat in the women who continued to exercise. The incidence of the water breaking well before the contractions start is significantly lower in women who continue exercise, as is the incidence of abnormalities in glucose tolerance. However, the incidence of late pregnancy complications that probably have their origins in abnormal placental development (pregnancy-induced hypertension, placental separation, and placenta previa) is about the same in exercisers and controls.

Poor uterine growth has been diagnosed in only four cases. Two occurred in women who were exercising and two in women who were physically active controls. Premature dilation of the cervix without premature labor has been diagnosed in 15 women (6 who exercised and 9 who did not). In each instance, they were placed on restricted activity and a drug to treat or prevent premature labor. On this regimen, four of the women who exercised and five of the controls went well beyond their due dates. They ultimately were induced for being *postdates*, suggesting that the initial concern that the cervix was dilating prematurely was erroneous or at least not clinically significant more than 50 percent of the time. The remaining two exercisers went into labor within 10 days of stopping the medicine at term, as did three of the controls. In these cases, the intervention may have been of value. Only one subject (a control) went into labor before term.

Beginning Regular Exercise During Pregnancy

Our experience in assessing the effect of starting exercise training programs on the incidence of pregnancy complications is still limited (about 80 women). However, we have yet to see any suggestion that our training regimen has any pronounced effects in this area one way or the other. To date we have had one case of premature rupture of the membranes leading to preterm birth and one case of postpartum depression. That's it.

Maternal Fitness and Physical Performance

All the studies that have examined indexes of fitness find that beginning or continuing a regular exercise regimen during pregnancy and lactation improves maternal fitness without identifiable risk (Clapp and Capeless 1991b; Collings, Curet, and Mullen 1983; Kulpa, White, and Visscher 1987; Sibley et al. 1981; South-Paul, Rajagopal, and Tenholder 1988; Wong and McKenzie 1987). Women who continue regular exercise throughout pregnancy and resume it postpartum experience about a 10-percent increase in their maximal aerobic capacity, even though their exercise volume is uniformly reduced by the added responsibilities of childcare. Women who continue but then stop do not achieve the same effect. Indeed, their maximal capacity falls a bit.

Women who start relatively low-volume exercise programs during pregnancy (20 minutes, three to five times a week, at a moderately hard level of perceived exertion) appear to increase their efficiency (improvement in the ratio between the increase in oxygen consumption and the increase in pulse rate) and time to fatigue; however, in our experience, they do not improve their maximal aerobic capacity. But women who start and maintain a higher volume training program throughout pregnancy (40 to 60 minutes, five times a week, at a moderately hard level of perceived exertion) demonstrate about a 10-percent improvement in their maximal aerobic capacity when we test them six weeks after the delivery.

Women who continue or start regular exercise during pregnancy improve fitness, and most improve performance as well.

The question of whether physical performance is improved by regular exercise during pregnancy is not totally resolved. There are two basic problems. First, like religion and politics, everyone with an interest has an opinion, but there is little definitive information. Second, no two subjects and no two training regimens are the same, so the outcome of the interaction between the pregnancy and the exercise regimen on performance will always be highly variable (Clapp 1996a). For example, on the one hand, I don't think anyone would disagree that the sedentary woman who increases her time to fatigue by 50 percent and reduces the ratio between her oxygen consumption and pulse rate by 20 percent has improved her performance. On the other hand, the national class distance runner who maintains her aerobic base but cuts back on her overall training regimen may be a different story. Chances are high that both her interval time and time over distance will increase during pregnancy.

Here's what's said on both sides of the question. First, many anecdotes from sport support the idea that the competitive performance of national class athletes who continue to train during and after pregnancy is enhanced after having a baby. Likewise, individual competitive performances in early and midpregnancy have produced many medals and personal bests. This suggests—but does not prove—that the changes in blood volume and hormonal levels during pregnancy may improve performance in track and field (Clapp and Capeless 1991b; Cohen et al. 1989; Higdon 1981). The same is true for competitive performance and maximal oxygen uptake after pregnancy (Clapp and Capeless 1991b; Villarosa 1985), suggesting that the combination of exercise and pregnancy has a greater training effect than that produced by training alone.

Second, several additional studies in fit, active women have identified changes that suggest a capacity for improved performance. They use less oxygen to complete standardized low-intensity treadmill exercise as pregnancy advances (Clapp 1989b; van Raaij et al. 1990). The ability to dissipate heat improves (Clapp 1991). The increases in cardiac volumes and decreased vascular resistance persist to some degree for at least one year postpartum, and maximal aerobic capacity increases (Clapp and Capeless 1991b; Clapp, Capeless, et al. 1995).

But, as noted earlier, many physically active women spontaneously decrease their exercise training volume in the latter third of pregnancy, which is undeniable evidence of a decrease in performance. The 15- to 25-percent increase in weight and abdominal protrusion do limit some aspects of performance—such as speed, balance, acceleration, and sudden lateral motion on a short-term basis (Carpenter et al. 1990; Clapp and Capeless 1991a, 1991b; Clapp, Wesley, and Sleamaker 1987; Cohen et al. 1989; Dale, Mullinax, and Bryan 1982; Lotgering et al. 1991).

Subtle Benefits

Some apparent benefits of exercise are very difficult to quantify because they either involve the personal opinion of the women or are impossible to test because many potentially confounding factors cannot be adequately controlled. Nevertheless, I highlight some of the differences observed in the attitudes of the women toward themselves, the pregnancy, and life in general. I also discuss several potential benefits including a decrease in one's susceptibility to the common cold and general respiratory infection, as well as an increase in one's energy level, or what I call *get up and go*.

Positive Attitude

One question we haven't been able to sort out fully is which is the cause and which is the effect: the exercise or the positive attitude? Are the women's positive attitudes the result of regular exercise, or, are women with these attitudes the ones who choose to exercise regularly? Most women who have exercised regularly for several years have a positive self-image about their appearance and physical capacity relative to their nonexercising peers. This positive attitude does not change during pregnancy and lactation *if* they continue to exercise. They maintain a positive self-image, feel extremely well, and are actually proud of the size of their bellies, and many feel the same way about their busts. The woman shown in figure 6.7 is a case in point. Anyone who doubts this is welcome to visit our exercise lab and observe and talk to the women we study. We have a *rogues' gallery* of photos taken in late pregnancy, which range all the way from conservative displays to bikini poses! They are equally proud of their physical abilities and the fact that they remain fit and ready for the challenge of labor.

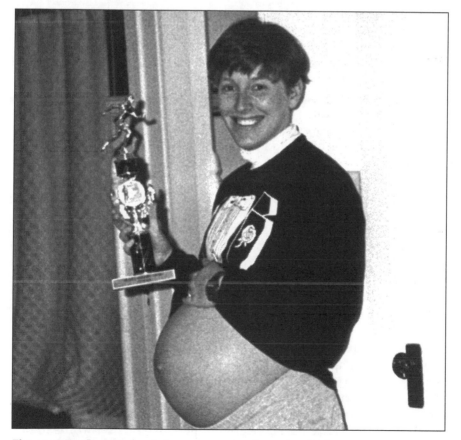

Figure 6.7   Positive body image—and a champion too!

This positive attitude is not the norm for the women who stop exercising during pregnancy. They begin to worry about their weight gain, appearance, and capabilities, especially if experiencing their first pregnancy. Many voice the concern that they will be unable to regain their prepregnancy look after the pregnancy.

Women who exercise regularly during pregnancy
maintain positive attitudes about themselves,
their pregnancies, and their upcoming
labor and delivery.

In my opinion, the most interesting group in our lab are the women like the one shown in figure 6.8 who have enrolled in the training program and been randomized either to maintain a high level of performance or to steadily increase their performance as pregnancy progresses. They feel so good about their appearance and capability in mid- and late pregnancy that, in many instances, we have to hold them back or they would exceed their assigned amount of exercise in the training protocol (although more exercise might increase benefit, it would ruin the study). The women who have been randomized to lower levels of performance have many of the same attitudes, but they are not held with the same intensity.

The women who continue to exercise during pregnancy also have strikingly positive attitudes about the pregnancy, labor, delivery, and lactation. The best way to describe their attitudes is they regard these events as a normal part of life and therefore take them in stride. They do not worry and fret or let these happenings interfere with other aspects of their lives to any great extent. If they have a question they ask, get the answer, and move on in a matter-of-fact way. In their view, pregnancy, birth, and lactation are fulfilling things they have wanted to experience, and now they're here to enjoy! To some extent these feelings are shared by women who continue to exercise then stop. The main difference appears to be that these women are not quite so self-assured, and worry and doubt occasionally creep in. By and large, the women who start exercising during pregnancy do so because they feel that it will be good for them and the pregnancy. Curiosity and delight intermixed with occasional concern are perhaps the best words to describe their attitude about their pregnancies.

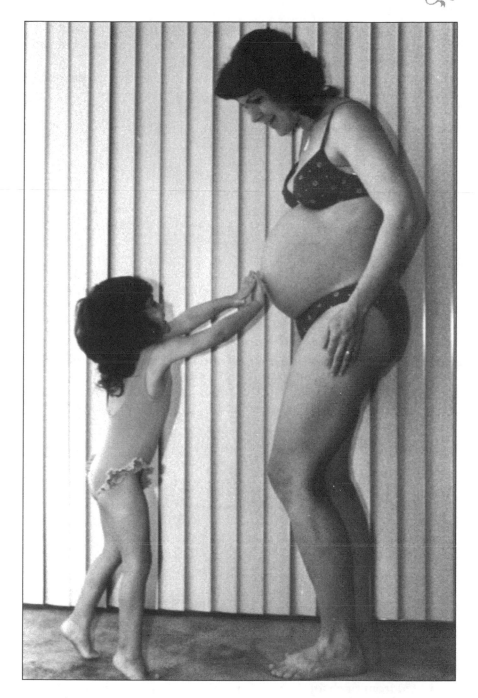

Figure 6.8 The joys of pregnancy—an inner becomes an outer!

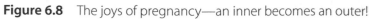

We see the same positive approach in the attitudes of the exercising women toward life in general. They get up in the morning feeling well and looking forward to the day, their jobs, the food they will eat, perhaps a little romance, and their exercise! They maintain their sense of humor and laugh about little unanticipated things that happen to them, their mates, and friends. Simply put, they seem to see the bright or humorous side to most things in their lives to the point where it sometimes becomes contagious. Unfortunately, the same cannot be said for the physically active controls.

Immune Function

We have been struck by the fact that most women we study stay healthy during pregnancy and lactation. The question is "Does the amount of exercise these women do improve their immune function or are they healthy to begin with?" What is clear right now is that the incidence of respiratory tract infection (colds, flu syndromes, sinusitis, and bronchitis) is much lower in the women who continue to exercise than in those who don't. Although we haven't studied this yet, we plan to, because regular exercise enhances immune function in nonpregnant individuals (Mackinnon 1992). Indeed, as upper respiratory infections are more common and more serious in pregnancy, this may represent another area in which the effect of regular exercise negates a potentially detrimental effect of pregnancy.

Energy Level

Closely tied in with the positive attitude shown by the women continuing exercise throughout pregnancy is that most women who continue regular exercise throughout pregnancy and lactation feel well and have impressive get up and go. By that I mean, pregnancy and lactation don't slow them down much. There is time for everything even though everything takes time. The best example of this comes in the period right after their first birth. Believe it or not, between 80 and 90 percent of the women who exercise are well enough organized so a two-hour return visit to the lab four or five days after the birth does not pose a problem for them. Although an equal percentage of the control women plan to complete the five-day evaluation before they give birth, only about half as many make it. Furthermore, the exercising women don't appear stressed when they arrive and already are comfortable being separated from the baby for an hour while a relative stranger evaluates his or her neurodevelopmental status. We cannot say the same for the majority of the controls.

Long-Term Outcome

We are only beginning to explore the question of women's long-term outcomes following exercise during pregnancy, but it is so important and the early information is so exciting that I thought I should end this chapter by sharing what we do know about the long-term effects of exercise during pregnancy on these women's general health, weight, fitness, and functional capacity.

> Women who exercise regularly during and after pregnancy improve their fitness, return to their prepregnancy weight, lose fat, and do not become injury-prone.

When we started these studies we thought that a quick look at the question of exercise in pregnancy would be all that was necessary. It turns out that nothing could be farther from the truth! Whenever we think we have definitively answered all the important questions, one of the women will ask another one or one of us gets a new idea. Long-term outcome for the women is one of those areas. Currently the two major questions are as follows:

- What effects does exercise during pregnancy have on a woman's fitness, weight, and long-term function?
- Does exercise during pregnancy leave the mother better off or worse off in the long run?

Fitness

Continuing to exercise during and after pregnancy has a training effect that is greater than what nonpregnant women attain with training alone over the same time interval (Clapp and Capeless 1991b). When studied one year after the birth, women who exercise throughout their pregnancies and maintain a regular exercise regimen after the birth routinely increase their maximum aerobic capacity by 5 to 10 percent, even though their training volumes are consistently lower than they were before becoming pregnant. In contrast, women who maintain a similar training regimen over the same two-year interval without getting pregnant fall off a bit. Thus, in a woman who is already fit, the combination of exercise and pregnancy gives her an edge that she would have had a hard time achieving without the addition of pregnancy.

Likewise, most of the women who have *begun* our progressive exercise regimen during pregnancy have maintained both the exercise and improved fitness after the birth. However, we cannot say with certainty that they are better off than they would have been with an equivalent training volume without the pregnancy.

Unfortunately, we have not seen this improved capacity reflected in better race times in many of the competitive women runners and cross-country skiers we have studied. In our experience, over 90 percent of the women have race times that are a little slower rather than a little faster after the birth. As their maximum aerobic capacities are higher, the reason for this appears to be that both training volume and motivation are lower after the baby is born. Finishing high up in the standings simply isn't as important anymore for most women. However, the women who are serious and continue to train at or above their prepregnancy level do better after the birth. Some say that it's improved focus, mental attitude, or a change in pain tolerance that makes a difference. Clearly, any of these could change as the result of the reproductive experience and make a real difference. Given the 1991 study (Clapp and Capeless 1991b), however, which showed a difference over time between women who experienced pregnancy and those who did not, my bias is that the training effect of pregnancy is the major factor in the improved performance of the motivated, competitive woman.

Body Weight and Composition

We've made several observations that suggest that most women who continue their exercise do not gain or retain the proverbial additional five pounds of fat with each pregnancy. As a matter of fact, the exact opposite appears to be true. As I discussed in chapter 2, combining exercise and pregnancy probably increases a woman's lean body mass (Little, Clapp, and Ridzon 1995). Moreover, most women who continue to exercise are back to their preconception weight by one year after the birth (Clapp and Capeless 1991b; Clapp, Simonian, et al. 1995). Also, women who exercise and who are planning their second child are leaner and lighter than those planning their first (Clapp and Little 1995). We also have had the opportunity to study more than 30 women who have continued to exercise through two (and 2 through three) pregnancies. On average, they are lighter and leaner before their second pregnancy than they were before their first.

Finally, we have weighed and interviewed a group of exercising and control women five years after the birth, and the weights of the exercising women are no different than they were before the first pregnancy (Clapp 1996b). Unfortunately, the same is not true for the controls. Although there are exceptions, most women who do not restart a regular exercise regimen after the delivery (whether they exercised during pregnancy or not) retain both weight and body fat over similar time intervals.

Functional Status

Our data collection is not yet complete in this area. However, what we have now indicates that regular exercise during pregnancy does not make a woman injury-prone later. There is no evidence that continuing regular exercise during pregnancy and lactation results in joint trauma or ligamentous laxity that only shows up a year or more after the birth. Continuing exercise throughout pregnancy appears to decrease the duration of postpartum urinary stress incontinence and signs and symptoms of the pelvic relaxation syndrome. Likewise, abdominal muscle tone and posture are well maintained. We don't have all the information we need on sexual function yet, but all indications are that intercourse is less frequent but often more satisfying as time goes on whether one exercises or not.

Summary

Current information indicates that fit women who continue to perform weight-bearing exercise throughout pregnancy and lactation at or above 50 percent of their prepregnancy levels gain less weight; deposit and retain less fat; feel better; have shorter, less complicated labors; and recover more rapidly than women who either stop or don't exercise. In addition, there have been no identifiable maternal ill effects from either exercise during the pregnancy or early resumption of exercise after the birth.

The findings are mixed in women who begin to exercise during pregnancy. The only consistent finding is that various indexes of fitness and well-being improve. The specifics of the exercise regimen appear to be very important if they are to provide the additional benefits related to weight gain, labor, and recovery. Our experience indicates that these women need to perform frequent, prolonged periods of weight-bearing exercise up to the time of delivery to obtain the maximum benefits.

Thus, at this point, all the information we've gathered indicates that both short- and long-term outcomes are much better in women who continue their regular exercise during and after pregnancy. Clearly, this is the case for fitness, weight stability, and the functional parameters. So, our view is that exercise during pregnancy and lactation is good for Mom. Now, what about Baby?

CHAPTER 7

Benefits of Maternal Exercise for the Baby

When we began our studies, most people intersted in the issue of exercise in pregnancy expressed the concern that the physiological demands of exercise might damage the unborn baby by increasing its temperature or depriving it of needed oxygen, glucose, or other nutrients. Because this is a difficult area to study, no one had attempted to determine if there were any objective findings to support this concern. Likewise, no one had attempted to determine if there was any objective evidence that regular exercise during the pregnancy benefited the baby during labor and after birth. The best that was available was that the Apgar Score—a gross measure of the baby's physical and mental condition—was not depressed in offspring of women who had exercised throughout their pregnancies.

This simply wasn't enough for me! I've always viewed the issue of fetal well-being as the central risk-benefit question that needs to be answered before one can comfortably advocate sustained, vigorous exercise for pregnant women. Therefore, each of my experiments has included one or more elements designed to address the issue of potential fetal risk or benefit. I've discussed many of these in chapters 2 through 5 already (miscarriage, congenital malformations, prematurity, heat stress with potential fetal damage, and so on).

You'll recall that we found no evidence of risk for the baby, but we didn't find much benefit either.

What follows is a discussion focusing on the additional information we've uncovered, that I interpret to mean that maternal exercise has several benefits for the unborn baby. I begin with some of the babies' responses to maternal exercise at various times during pregnancy then move to evidence suggesting that the babies are in better condition at the start of labor and tolerate the stresses of labor better if their mothers exercised during pregnancy. Then, I discuss information indicating that these babies have a better growth and development pattern in utero than babies whose mothers did not exercise. Finally, I discuss some information that helped us understand why the babies born of exercising women are perhaps better off than those born of the physically active controls, and then end with the results of some of our long-term morphometric and neurodevelopmental follow-up studies of the offspring.

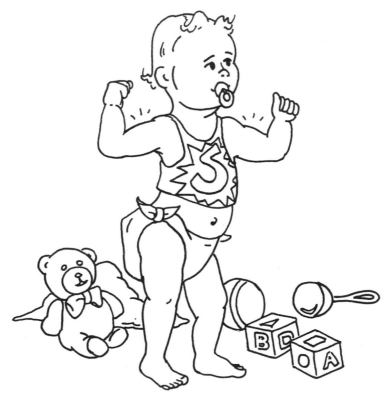

Superbaby!

Baby's Physical Responses to Maternal Exercise

The things that we looked at first in our studies included the baby's heart rate, bowel function, and physical activity in response to maternal exercise. All indicate that regular maternal exercise improves the baby's ability to deal effectively with the intermittent reductions in uterine blood flow and oxygen delivery that are a part of everyday life. This physiological benefit has real survival value for the baby because it provides additional protection when unanticipated maternal stresses occur, specifically during serious traumatic injury, other medical emergencies, and when complications arise during labor.

Fetal Heart Rate Response

Many investigators had looked at what effect exercise had on fetal heart rate before we did, but their findings were contradictory. No one, including us, knew what to make of these findings (Artal, Rutherford, et al. 1986; Carpenter et al. 1988; Clapp, Little, and Capeless 1993; Collings, Curet, and Mullen 1983; Wolfe and Mottola 1993). In most early studies, fetal heart rate was unchanged, in a few it went up, and, in an occasional subject, it went down. Again, the variable results suggested that some aspect of either the exercise regimens or the women studied would explain the different responses others had seen. So we decided to see if the fetal heart rate response was related to the various components of exercise (type, intensity, duration), characteristics of the woman (her health and fitness level), or perhaps to something about the pregnancy (healthy, early in the pregnancy, or late). Since that time, we have measured the fetal heart rate before, during, and after exercise in many women under different circumstances (Clapp 1985a; Clapp, Little, and Capeless 1993; Clapp, Tomaselli, et al. 1996).

The first thing we noted was that in almost 100 percent of the women the fetal heart rate went up during and immediately after the exercise. This indicated that the baby was probably experiencing mild stress during the exercise, which caused a reflex increase in heart rate. So, at least for the babies of the several hundred athletic women we have studied, the *normal* or usual response is an increase in heart rate during exercise that gradually returns to the preexercise baseline rate once the exercise session ends.

We found that many components of the exercise did make a difference in the heart rate response.

- The *duration* of the exercise was important. The exercise had to be continued for at least 10 minutes to see a consistent fetal heart rate response. This explained why many investigators saw little or nothing, because the exercise periods they used were less than this 10-minute threshold. All other things being equal, the longer the woman exercised beyond 10 minutes, the greater the increase in the fetal heart rate. It was like the creep upward you see in anyone's heart rate when they continue to exercise for a protracted time. This was consistent with the stress theory mentioned.

- The *type* of exercise was important as well. Activities requiring the woman to use a large fraction of her muscle mass to move her weight against gravity (aerobics, running, stair stepping, versa climber, cross-country skiing, and the like) resulted in a greater increase than those that didn't (swimming, biking, rowing, riding, and the like). This finding coupled with the finding that duration made a difference gave us an important clue. Namely, the trigger for the increase in the baby's heart rate was probably a fall in uterine blood flow, because using more muscle mass and exercising longer intensify the need for flow redistribution away from the internal organs to supply the exercising muscle. When uterine blood flow falls, so does the oxygen tension in the baby's blood. Special cells in the baby's blood vessels sense this change and initiate a stress response in the baby to compensate for the fall in oxygen tension.

- Exercise *intensity* is also a factor. To be sure that our interpretation was correct, we also looked at whether the fetal heart rate response to exercise increased when the mother worked harder, and it did. The harder a woman works, the greater the fall in uterine blood flow and the bigger the increase in the baby's heart rate.

- Finally, we examined whether the fetal heart rate response increased as the baby's *nervous system* became more mature. If our interpretation was right, then the increase in heart rate should be greater as delivery time came closer, and it was.

The normal response of a fetus to sustained exercise
is an increase in heart rate.

So it seemed clear that the magnitude of the increase in fetal heart rate varied directly with the magnitude of the stress that the baby was experiencing. This raised the question of how much stress was normal and how much was too much.

Determining the Safe Upper Limit of Stress

As a first step, we used an ultrasound technique to determine whether the stress was enough to cause the baby to increase its blood flow to the brain, and it was. Although this is a normal protective response, the fact that it occurred was bothersome and suggested that there was an upper limit above which there might be some risk. So we looked at other things to decide what would be a safe upper limit.

Fetal Bowel Function

We began by looking to see if the baby was stressed enough to lose control and move its bowels in utero. The baby is no different from you or me; when he gets stressed the amount of oxygenated blood that goes to the intestines drops to low levels, which stimulates the bowels to move. The material that a baby passes is called meconium, and, because it stains the fluid and membranes surrounding the baby a dark green color, it can be easily detected during labor when these membranes break.

So we took a close look at the babies of a group of women who exercised at a very high level of perceived exertion or for an extended duration or both in the last few weeks before delivery. We looked to see if those fetuses whose heart rates increased more than 25 beats per minute during maternal exercise also had meconium staining of their fluid when they were delivered. They didn't, indicating that an increase in fetal heart rate as high as 25 to 35 beats per minute above the preexercise rate was probably OK, as it did not drop oxygen levels low enough to stimulate the baby to move its bowels.

Fetal Breathing and Activity

Next we looked at the baby's breathing and activity during exercise. Remember, even before they're born, babies are a lot like you and me. When they don't feel well, they stop moving, and when they aren't getting enough oxygen, they make gasping movements that we can see with ultrasound. So we observed whether exercise had any effect. We never saw any gasps, but initially we noted that almost 100 percent of babies were quiet and did not make breathing motions for several minutes after their mothers stopped exercising. However, when we compared the babies' physical activity and breathing motions for the 20 minutes before exercise to those for the 20 minutes after exercise, the breathing movements were slightly decreased and physical activity was unchanged. If we compared the babies' shoulder activity after a rest to that after exercise, there was actually more activity after exercise. As maternal exercise did not produce changes in fetal breathing and activity patterns that are characteristic of insufficient oxygen, we concluded that the increases in the babies' heart rates were a normal stress response to the exercise, rather than a change produced by a significant decrease in oxygen availability (Hatoum et al. 1997).

Drop in Fetal Heart Rate

We've talked a lot about the baby's heart rate going up during and after exercise, but another possibility is that it could go down. It is important to recognize this heart rate response and understand what it means in case it happens. It has been known for some time that a sudden severe lack of oxygen causes the baby's heart rate to fall dramatically and stay low until oxygen availability improves. Therefore, although there are other things that can cause the baby's heart rate to fall (pressure on the umbilical cord or on the baby's head are two common ones), a sustained (more than a 20-second) drop in the baby's heart rate of 20 beats per minute or more during or after exercise should be interpreted as a serious lack of oxygen until proven otherwise.

Does this ever happen? Of course it does. There are several reports in the literature indicating that this fetal heart rate response to maternal exercise occurs somewhere between 15 and 20 percent of the time (Artal, Rutherford, et al. 1986; Carpenter et al. 1988; Wolfe and Mottola 1993). However, this response is usually observed when the investigators exercise relatively unfit women and have them increase their exercise intensity rapidly to the maximal level they can stand. As far as I'm concerned, this means that very strenuous exercise in this type of woman can cause uterine blood flow to fall far enough to create a serious lack of oxygen in the baby. Whether this happens when fit women exercise to their maximal level is unknown because the experiment has not been done, but we haven't seen it in the fit women we've studied who exercise at or above 85 percent of their maximum capacity. Does this fetal heart rate response to exercise ever occur in fit women? Yes it does, but it is rare. We have monitored well over 2,000 exercise sessions and seen it twice. In both cases, it happened near the time of delivery when the baby's head was already down in the mother's pelvis. Both women continued to exercise and delivered soon after. Neither baby had problems during labor and their amniotic fluid was clear. Therefore, we think that the fall in their heart rates during exercise was probably not caused by oxygen lack, but rather from pressure on their heads from the mother's pelvic structures.

Interpreting These Responses

The fact that the baby's heart rate goes up and not down means that the adaptations occurring with regular exercise make it possible for him or her to fully adjust to significant decreases in oxygen delivery without developing oxygen deficiency in the tissues of the heart. Likewise, the fact that strenuous or prolonged exercise near the time of delivery does not cause the baby to move its bowels in utero means that oxygen delivery to the intestines is not severely compromised. The fact that the baby's breathing motions and physical activity remain normal means that oxygen delivery to the brain and muscle is maintained as well. Thus, the baby of the exercising mother is probably much better prepared to deal with potential problems than the baby of a more sedentary woman. One of those potential problems is labor, and we'll look at that next.

A word about what to do if the baby's heart rate goes up very high (over 180 beats per minute), falls more than 20 beats per minute, or the baby stays quiet for a long time after exercise (more than 30 minutes). These fetal responses are rarely seen in healthy women with uncomplicated pregnancies. So, if one does occur interpret it as a valuable warning sign and obtain further medical evaluation. Acutely, the woman should lie down on her left side, drink fluids, and have the baby's heart rate and activity monitored. The baby's heart rate and activity should promptly return to their baseline levels. Then notify the doctor. Until proven otherwise, assume that any of these responses means that some link in the woman's oxygen delivery system (lungs, blood flow, placental function, and so on) may not be working properly. She should not stress her system with exercise again until this has been ruled out or the cause has been identified and any problem corrected.

You may ask the following:

"How will I know if this happens?"

"What can I do to check the baby's response?"

You won't know unless the baby's heart rate is monitored periodically or specific attention is paid to the baby's activity after exercise. Many women choose to check this regularly because it's reassuring to feel the baby move. Checking the baby's heart rate requires special equipment and training, but with practice, a woman can learn to do it herself. Based on our experiences, though, I don't recommend that a healthy woman with a normal pregnancy do it , pp. unless she falls into one of the special categories we discuss in chapter 8, pp. 126-128.

In mid- and late pregnancy, a fall in the baby's heart rate
or no kicking for 30 minutes after exercise are two valuable
warning signs to pregnant women and health fitness
personnel that the woman should see her doctor and
not exercise again until the situation is clarified.

Baby's Condition During Labor

If the baby of the exercising woman is *tougher*, then there should be big
differences detectable at the onset of labor and in his or her response
to labor. There should be less evidence of diminished reserve at the
onset of labor, and the baby's heart rate patterns should be more stable
during labor. Its condition at birth and ability to adapt to life outside
the uterus should be better as well.

Beginning of Labor

In our study, only 4 out of more than 250 babies carried by exercising
women worried the doctors at the start of labor. This is a very low
incidence (1 to 2 percent) for obstetrical concern and was much less
than that in either the nonexercising, physically active controls (15 cases,
or about 5 percent) or in the women who exercised then stopped (8
cases, or about 10 percent). But 2 cases in the exercise group caused
concern due to a decreased amount of amniotic fluid. This occurred
five times in the nonexercising, physically active controls and twice in
the women who stopped exercise in midpregnancy. Most other cases
were related to concerns that the baby was too big or the women had
gone too far past their due dates (one in the exercise group, seven in
the others). There were several cases of serious growth restriction (one
in the exercise group and three in the controls), maternal high blood
pressure, and vaginal bleeding. While the differences in the incidence
of these complications in all the groups are too low to be statistically
significant, the slightly lower frequency in the exercise group suggests
that the babies of the exercising women may well be in better condition at the beginning of labor.

Next, we measured the levels of erythropoietin (a hormone) in the
amniotic fluid early in labor in each exercising woman to be very sure
that exercise in late pregnancy didn't compromise the baby's oxygen

supply. Erythropoietin is the hormone released when oxygen levels in the body get low, and it stimulates the body to make more red blood cells to improve oxygen delivery. It's the hormone that increases the number of red blood cells in people who live at high altitude or in people who have serious lung disease. It also increases in babies who have low levels of oxygen before birth and thus is a very sensitive marker for oxygen lack prior to birth. After erythropoietin does its job, it is excreted by the kidneys, and for the unborn baby this means that it ends up in the surrounding fluid where it hangs around for some time. So, we collected a sample of the fluid surrounding each baby whose mother exercised until delivery and each baby whose mother didn't exercise in late pregnancy and compared them (Clapp, Little, et al. 1995). As you might expect, the levels of erythropoietin weren't any higher and actually tended to be lower in the exercise group indicating that, if anything, these babies had experienced less oxygen lack than the controls.

During Labor

The first thing we looked at during labor was the babies' heart rate responses to the contractions of labor. We found evidence that the babies of the women who continued to exercise tolerated the stress of the contractions much better than either the controls or the women who stopped exercise well before term. The incidence of the doctor, nurse, or midwife becoming concerned about the baby's condition was less than half that in the controls. Next, we looked to see whether the mother's exercise had caused the baby to get tangled in the umbilical cord—which often causes a problem when the cord tightens as the baby gets lower in the birth canal late in labor. Again, we were pleasantly surprised. The incidence of cord entanglement hadn't increased, rather, it significantly decreased. We looked at the meconium issue to see how many babies were stressed enough to move their bowels during labor, and again the number was much lower in the babies of the exercising moms.

As a final check, we drew blood samples from the umbilical cords of the babies of the exercising moms and the controls at the time of birth and measured several things. First, the levels of erythropoietin stayed low, indicating that oxygen availability was adequate during labor. Second, the percentages of red cells in the blood from babies of the exercising moms were lower, indicating that the babies had been relatively stress-free for some time. The same was true for measurements of acid accumulation in the blood. So, all the evidence indicated that the babies of the exercising moms were indeed tougher, in that the usual stresses of late pregnancy and labor didn't produce as many warning signs of difficulty requiring attention during labor.

Neonatal Condition

Once the babies were born, we examined how they did in the first few days after birth to see how well they were prepared for the transition out of the womb. Because the babies of the exercising moms weren't as fat, we looked to see if they had trouble maintaining their body temperature; they didn't. They had no difficulty with early weight loss and regained their birth weight rapidly. We checked their blood glucose levels to see if they were normal, and they were fine. To date, only four cases of low blood sugar have occurred, and they all have been in babies born of control women or women who stopped exercise. I interpret this to mean that the lean babies born of women who exercise are not starved and are metabolically normal. Thus, even though the babies of exercising moms are lighter and leaner, they show none of the signs in the immediate newborn period that usually accompany growth retardation. This suggests that these babies are the normal ones, and the bigger, fatter babies born of the control women are overgrown.

> The newborns of women who exercise don't have trouble
> with the transition to life outside the uterus and
> tend to be alert and easy to care for.

The next thing we noticed was that many exercising moms told us their babies were much easier to care for than they had expected. They proudly told us that their babies slept through the night early on, didn't have colic, and so on. It appeared that these babies might have different personality characteristics. So, to see if this was the case, we began a blind evaluation of the babies' personalities and neurodevelopment five days after birth. The preliminary findings (Clapp, Simonian, et al. 1995) indicate that the mothers' impressions were right on. On average, the babies born of the women who continued to exercise throughout pregnancy do better in two areas:

- They respond readily to things in their environment.
- They readily self-quiet when they are disturbed and need much less consolation from others.

Both characteristics suggest that they are more mature at birth, and, as shown in figure 7.1, this makes them what I call *easy keepers* for the parents.

Why Babies Benefit From Maternal Exercise

Again we must ask "Why?" Why should regular exercise result in a tougher baby who does better in the transition to life outside the womb and who may do better later on? We don't have all the answers to this intriguing question, but we have several good guesses.

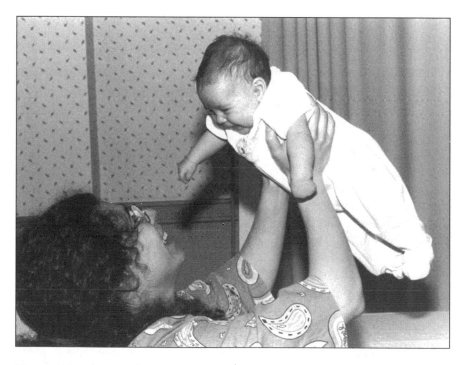

Figure 7.1   An *easy keeper*.

Value of Intermittent Stress and Stimuli

There is evidence indicating that all biological systems respond and are changed by stresses and stimuli. This is true of development during infancy, childhood, adolescence, and adulthood. Indeed, the functional changes caused by the stimuli and stresses of exercise training in adults are a good example of this. Another is the development of sight, hearing, and speech. Without impressions on the retina of the eye, the optical area of the brain does not develop properly. The same is true for sound and the auditory pathways in the brain. Anyone who has had a child knows the value of conversation in speech development.

> Sound and vibratory stimuli before birth may accelerate the development of the baby's brain.

Perhaps we should ask ourselves why it should be any different before birth. When a woman exercises, she creates stimuli that might alter development and maturation of the baby in a positive way. First, there are the intermittent changes in the delivery of fuel and oxygen that we've talked about. Perhaps that makes the baby and its placenta more efficient in ways we haven't uncovered yet. Then, there is the intermittent increase in sound and vibration stimuli. It's clear that the baby can hear a lot of what goes on in the mother's environment. Perhaps, this speeds development and starts to mature many pathways in the brain. Indeed, there are a host of people who believe that playing classical music as well as talking and reading to the baby before it is born will make it a more relaxed infant and help its development after birth. Then, there are the intermittent changes in heart rate, temperature, and other things as well. Perhaps they improve the developmental capacity of the heart, the thermoregulatory system, and who knows what else. We'll have to wait until these kids are older to test them and see.

Specific Stimulus Responses

I think you'll agree that many things we have identified to date support this stimulus-response explanation of exercise's effects on the fetus, newborn, and infant. The extra increase in maternal blood volume, the improved growth and function of the placenta, and the increased ability to dissipate heat are three clear maternal examples of a response to the stimuli of exercise and pregnancy. Although we haven't examined the babies directly, the responses that we have been able to measure hint that their toughness is not simply a result of the changes that exercise induces in the mother. For example, the volume of the blood vessels on the baby's side of the placenta is increased, and the percentage of the blood that is comprised of red cells is decreased in blood obtained from the umbilical cord at birth. Both these observations suggest that the babies born to exercising mothers have increased blood volumes. This may help the baby maintain blood flows to all tissues when it is stressed, exactly like it does in the mother. Likewise, the changes in behavior before and after birth suggest that the multiple stimuli maternal exercise generates have initiated adaptations that may prove valuable later in life. Indeed, as you will see from the next few paragraphs, we already have some good hints that this is the case.

Long-Term Outcome

One major difficulty for a midwife or a doctor who practices obstetrics is deciding the best way to manage a problem. The reason it's difficult is that often there is little or no follow-up information available. So there is no way for them to know which method of management results in the best long-term outcome for the baby.

All aspects of growth and development after birth in babies
from exercising mothers are equal to or better than
those observed in the control offspring.

For this reason, we thought that the story would be incomplete without additional information on long-term outcome. Clearly the final word about the safety and benefits of exercise during pregnancy rests on how the offspring turn out.

- Will they be fat or thin?
- Will they be ahead or behind their peers developmentally?
- Will there be any evidence of damage that doesn't show up until later or will they be *superstars* later on?

The only way to tell is to track these babies down, test them, and see. So we sat down with a group of psychologists to determine what the best time in life is to see how these kids turned out. The answer was the fourth grade or later. Well, I wasn't sure I'd still be around if we waited that long. So we decided to check a group of them in detail at one year of age and another group at the next best time, right before they started formal education (age five).

One Year of Age

To date we've managed to evaluate almost 100 offspring at one year of age, and the results favor the offspring of the women who continued to exercise throughout pregnancy. There are no differences in the physical configuration of the offspring in the two groups. They weigh the same, are the same height, have the same circumferential measurements and the same amount of fat. This last one surprised us, but it probably is because of the time when we chose to make the measurements. All babies get fat until they learn to walk, then many of them thin out. Unfortunately for us, most babies are just starting to walk at one year of age.

It looks as if babies born of exercising women do better on standardized intelligence tests at one year of age. To date, they have done significantly better on the standardized Bayley Test of Infant Development than the offspring of the physically active controls. Their mental performance is slightly but significantly better, and their physical performance is better as well.

Five Years of Age

We completed this initial series of evaluations in the offspring at age five, and the findings were exciting (Clapp 1996b). It's important to point out that we didn't evaluate every baby because we were concerned that many factors other than exercise might confuse the issue. Instead, we selected 20 babies born of women who exercised vigorously throughout pregnancy and who had no detectable problems during pregnancy, labor, delivery, infancy, or childhood. We compared their growth and development to that of 20 similar babies born of the women who were physically active controls. In addition, we carefully matched them for multiple pre- and postnatal factors that influence growth and development. For example, we matched them for parental weight, height, education, and socioeconomic status. We matched them for their mother's physical activity after the birth and working outside the home, as well as sex, birth order, general health, breast-feeding, estimated caloric intake, family recreation profile, and type of childcare. Then, within a month of their fifth birthday, I measured their weight, height, and so on, and a trained psychologist, who didn't know who exercised and who didn't, did a detailed two-day evaluation of their mental and physical capacities. All the findings indicate that exercise during pregnancy does no harm and may improve long-term outcome for the baby.

- There were no differences in height, limb lengths, or head and chest circumferences between the offspring of the women who exercised and those who didn't.
- The offspring of the women who exercised were not only less fat at birth but still weighed a little less and were not as fat as the offspring of the physically active controls.
- There were no differences noted between the two groups in their academic readiness skills (reading and math), physical coordination, dexterity, or visual-motor integration.
- The offspring of the women who exercised scored much higher on tests of general intelligence and oral language skills than the offspring of the physically active controls.

So the babies who were lean at birth grew normally throughout infancy and childhood but stayed lean. If this persists, it may have long-term benefit because this physical profile has a reduced risk for cardiovascular and metabolic diseases later in life.

Likewise, we could find no evidence that either mental or motor development was compromised by the mother exercising during the pregnancy. In fact, it appears that they are better in several areas. However, the possibility exists that this finding is the result of some unrecognized aspect of the child's life that we didn't control for, so we have decided to do three additional things, which are currently under way. First, examine these kids again when they are older. Second, evaluate the growth, general intelligence, and oral language skills of all the current offspring as they turn five. Third, evaluate all the offspring at one year of age to rule out any possible confounders related to differences in environmental circumstances between one and five years of age. At present, the only one of these that we have enough information to discuss are the findings we presented earlier in this chapter of the children at one year of age. In any case, the findings to date should be reassuring to both women who plan to continue to exercise during pregnancy and those who care for them.

Summary

Despite concerns that sustained, vigorous, maternal exercise would harm the unborn baby and compromise long-term outcome, everywhere we have looked we have found evidence suggesting that maternal exercise during pregnancy has both short- and long-term benefits for the fetus in utero. The evidence for this opinion is broad. It includes the baby's heart rate and behavioral responses to a wide range of exercise programs, coupled with biochemical and clinical evidence that these babies tolerate the stresses of late pregnancy, labor, and delivery better than the babies of the control women. It includes the findings of studies that have examined placental growth and function during pregnancy, as well as the assessment of morphometric and behavioral outcome near the time of birth, in infancy, and early childhood. These studies have shown that the offspring of exercising women have advantages in many areas and have not identified any evidence of deficit. In truth, we have yet to find any short- or long-term problem that has arisen because a woman continues to exercise during pregnancy and lactation. That being the case, it's time to turn our attention to how to develop a holistic, individualized exercise program for each phase of the reproductive process. The next chapter starts that part of the book by formulating some principles for exercise prescription during pregnancy and lactation.

PART III

Exercise Prescription and Monitoring

Part III is designed to be used by both physically active women and health care and health fitness providers. It provides both with the necessary information to develop an individualized exercise program for use during pregnancy and lactation and can be used by either the woman herself or in conjunction with a health care or health fitness provider. Chapter 8 answers the broad questions (such as, who does and who doesn't need an exercise prescription, and contraindications to exercise), develops general principles, and stresses the common sense themes applied in the chapters that follow. Chapters 9, 10, and 11 each focus on the specifics of exercise prescription at conception and early pregnancy, later in pregnancy, and after the birth. These chapters begin by reviewing the pertinent physiological events occurring at that time and then go on to address the specific needs of beginner, recreational, and competitive athletes separately.

I stress a common sense, flexible approach throughout. Finally, in order to be sure that the exercise prescriptions will truly be individualized, I specifically avoid recommending a set type, number, or pattern of exercises to be performed. Instead, I use a holistic approach that addresses the educational, interactive, instructional, safety, and monitoring aspects of the program and only give general advice about the exercise regimen itself (types, frequency, volume, and so on). However, every section of each chapter details how to determine how much exercise is enough for both the woman and the pregnancy and addresses specific dos and don'ts for each group (beginner, recreational, and competitive athletes) during the different phases of the reproductive process.

CHAPTER 8

Principles for Exercise Prescription

This chapter uses the information from the first two parts to establish a set of principles to use when developing an effective exercise prescription during each phase of the reproductive process. You'll notice three distinct themes throughout this chapter:

1. The *approach to exercise prescription* should be the same for women who are either trying to get pregnant, pregnant, recovering from the birth, or lactating, as it is for nonpregnant women who are not planning a pregnancy in the near future.

2. A holistic approach to exercise is valuable to the individual because it brings balance and understanding to the relationships among a woman's life, her exercise regimen, and her pregnancy.

3. Most genuinely healthy noncompetitive women who exercise to appetite for relaxation and fun probably don't need a new exercise prescription simply because they're planning pregnancy. They can continue with their regular exercise regimen throughout pregnancy without a specific prescription as long as no major changes in exercise volume are planned.

First and foremost, when developing an individualized exercise program, it's important to remember that the exercise regimen does not exist in a vacuum. No one should treat it as a goal in itself. Indeed, a new exercise program probably isn't necessary for most women who are already exercising recreationally simply because they are or wish to become pregnant. For example, a fit, healthy pregnant woman who continues to jog or do aerobics and other health club activities three times a week to stay fit probably doesn't need a new exercise prescription, *unless* she develops a problem or decides she wants to increase her exercise load to improve her fitness and performance. Likewise, if a woman training for a marathon experiences an unanticipated pregnancy and stops training for an upcoming marathon, she doesn't necessarily need an exercise prescription; but if she wants to continue to train for the marathon, she will need one.

In any case, if it is deemed necessary to develop a new exercise program for pregnancy, approach it as only one piece of the daily puzzle that makes up a pregnant woman's life, and then design it to fit.

Second, the exercise prescription should include many things in addition to the exercise itself. These include the following:

Education	Observation
Interaction	Safety
Instruction	Monitoring

The educational component provides perspective, and the interactive component should ensure that the exercise program matches the individual's exercise goals and also should take into account the inevitable changes that will occur in a woman's life as she passes through the various phases of pregnancy and lactation. The instructional and observational components of the exercise program can help a woman exercise safely and prevent problems with biomechanics. Finally, develop a plan to monitor the progress of *both* the exercise regimen *and* the pregnancy so that neither is compromised. Now let's talk about some of the details involved in developing an individualized exercise program immediately before, during, or after pregnancy.

Who Needs an Exercise Prescription?

How do you decide who does and who doesn't need her exercise program reviewed or modified during the reproductive process? There are basically two key points to remember:

1. What is the level of motivation for exercise?
2. What are the current health or exercise habits and do they place the woman or pregnancy at risk?

If an individual is not motivated toward new or different goals that require a change in her exercise regimen, then there is no need for her to modify her exercise routine simply because she's contemplating pregnancy. Likewise, healthy women whose exercise regimens are well established and low risk or involve intermittent low-intensity activity can continue to exercise at that level without a change in their exercise program. Most women who walk or jog regularly, go to the health club two or three times a week, or hike, swim, play golf, play tennis, or the like on the weekends fall into this category. Even women who are healthy recreational athletes (who exercise every day of the week) can continue with their exercise program without changing it for the pregnancy. Unfortunately, there is no exact frequency, duration, or intensity in an exercise program defining where a woman should draw the line. Still, the answers to two simple questions before pregnancy should establish whether she needs to review or modify her exercise program for pregnancy:

1. Does she compete on a regular basis (six or more times per year)? If the answer is "yes" her exercise program needs to be reviewed and perhaps modified.

2. Are her periods consistently regular (occurring every 25 to 35 days)? If the answer is "no," then there may be a problem with either ovulation or the length of the luteal phase. As either or both could interfere with successful conception, her current exercise program needs to be reviewed and perhaps modified.

There are four groups of women who definitely will benefit from a detailed evaluation of and recommendations for their exercise program during the reproductive process.

1. Women who want to *begin* an exercise program. It's either their first exercise program or they haven't been successful sticking to an exercise program in the past. In these cases, the cardinal rule in developing a successful and appropriate exercise program is ongoing motivation and incentive.

2. Competitive athletes who wish to have a baby *and* maintain or improve their performance at the same time. The cardinal rule in this group is to be sure that the depth and detail of all the nonexercise aspects of the program match the level of exercise performance that the athlete desires. For example, the approach to monitoring fetal wellbeing in a competitive athlete should involve frequent measurements of fetal heart rate responses, maternal temperature, fetal activity patterns, maternal blood glucose levels, and fetal growth rather than

simply a few questions and an abdominal measurement. In these cases, it is important to follow the adage "An ounce of prevention is worth a pound of cure." Our limited experience with competitive athletes coupled with the limited knowledge in this area leads us to recommend that all competitive athletes should consult with a health fitness professional for help in designing a holistic program to follow during the time of conception, pregnancy, and lactation. If available, I recommend that competitive athletes may also explore the possibility of volunteering as study subjects for any research protocols dealing with exercise in pregnancy that are ongoing in their local areas.

A competitive athlete considering pregnancy should always involve one or more health fitness professionals in developing and monitoring an individualized training plan that will fulfill both her training and reproductive needs throughout conception, pregnancy, and lactation.

---

3. Recreational athletes who become *motivated* to go further than they feel they can go on their own. In this case, the cardinal rule is education coupled with careful monitoring and a progressive upregulation of training volume. Remember that it is clear that success is tightly linked to progress, and progress is best assessed by detailed, periodic evaluations of performance.

4. Women who have *underlying disease* that may be improved or worsened by regular exercise. Although a detailed discussion of exercise prescription for this group is beyond the scope of this book, the cardinal rule is always use a team approach. Make sure that there is input as well as follow-up from all appropriate sources. Whether this is you or someone you're working with, meet face to face with the physician or physicians involved regularly, especially if there are underlying orthopedic, endocrine, pulmonary, or cardiovascular problems.

The Right Amount of Exercise

The next two obvious questions are as follows:

1. How much exercise is enough to obtain the positive effects we've talked about?
2. Is there a safe upper limit?

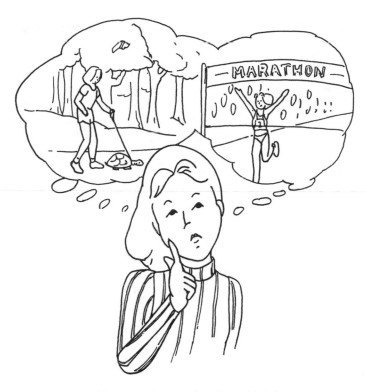

How much exercise should I do?

The answers to both are essential for designing safe and effective training programs. These questions are more complicated than they look, however, because they encompass a subset of questions you must answer before deciding what range of exercise is right for a specific individual during pregnancy and lactation. Therefore, I begin by discussing the subset of questions, then use that information to answer how to decide what's too much exercise, what's too little, and what's right. In terms of the risks and benefits to mother and baby, the subset includes many of the following questions:

- Is early pregnancy a better time to exercise than late pregnancy?
- Do all types of exercise provide the same benefits?
- Does it matter if the effort involved is light, medium, or hard?
- Is 20 minutes three times a week enough? Is 60 to 90 minutes every day overdoing it?

In the next few paragraphs I review the findings in these areas and answer these and other questions one at a time.

Exercise at Different Times During Pregnancy

At the outset, it's important to remember that the information from the previous chapters indicates that regular weight-bearing exercise during pregnancy and lactation does not appear to be harmful to the mother or baby. Rather, it appears to be helpful, and, as different things are going on in early and late pregnancy (see chapter 2), it makes sense that exercise at different times during pregnancy and lactation should have beneficial effects on different aspects of the pregnancy. So, it helps to view exercise during pregnancy and lactation as a lifestyle factor that can improve pregnancy outcome by varying the exercise regimen at different points in the pregnancy.

Regular exercise in early and midpregnancy often improves many bothersome symptoms (fatigue, nausea, and so forth) and enhances both maternal adaptations and placental growth and functional capacity. The latter introduces an additional margin of safety, paving the way for the baby's growth. Continuing regular exercise throughout late pregnancy maintains many aspects of maternal fitness. If the intensity level is appropriate, it also limits maternal weight gain and fat deposition in both mother and baby and has many positive effects on the course and outcome of labor.

The benefits of exercise are different in early and late pregnancy. Early pregnancy exercise improves the growth of the baby and decreases maternal symptoms. Late pregnancy exercise maintains fitness, limits weight gain, and shortens labor.

So, the question becomes "What is the right amount of exercise to accomplish each goal for the exercise program and the pregnancy at different times during the reproductive process?" To answer this question, evaluate the current status of the exercise program, fitness level, and the current stage of pregnancy. Then set specific, realistic goals in all areas and develop a program that will achieve them without endangering the reproductive process. For example, if a healthy woman has exercised regularly all along, she can do at least as much as usual while attempting pregnancy and at any time during pregnancy and lactation. Thus, the right amount of exercise for her at different times will depend on her fitness goals and what she wants in terms of maternal and fetal benefits. If a woman is beginning to exercise regularly for the first time, it won't take a lot of exercise to make her feel good and improve the growth of her placenta and baby. It will, however, take a lot more in mid- and late pregnancy to modify weight gain and shorten labor. The safe upper limit for exercise performance appears to be dictated by a woman's physical condition at the start and the health of the pregnancy. In a healthy woman experiencing a normal pregnancy, the problem usually is not what the baby can safely tolerate, but what the woman can safely tolerate without developing the symptoms of overtraining. I discuss this more later.

Type of Exercise

The fact that specific forms of exercise improve various aspects of fitness suggests that the type of exercise should make a difference in its ability to enhance the physiological adaptations to pregnancy. For example, central cardiovascular, thermal, and systemic metabolic responses to training are most rapidly obtained by performing sustained weight-bearing activity, using a large fraction of an individual's muscle mass (running, aerobics, and cross-country skiing versus stationary cycling, hiking, racquet and ball sports, or weight training). As these systemic responses are the adaptations that complement those of pregnancy, these forms of exercise are probably superior. One reason some exercise regimens have little or no effect on outcome whereas others have a lot is probably partially due to differences in the physiological effects of the types of exercise performed. So, weight-bearing activities are probably the best.

Regular, sustained, weight-bearing exercise is the best type of exercise for pregnant women because it clearly complements the adaptations to pregnancy. However, the proper frequency, duration, and intensity will vary from woman to woman.

The types of exercise a woman chooses should match the goals of her training program as well as her lifestyle. It is important for beginners to find the exercise fun and easy to do. The same is true for the recreational or not-so-serious athlete. Uncertainty, awkwardness, and

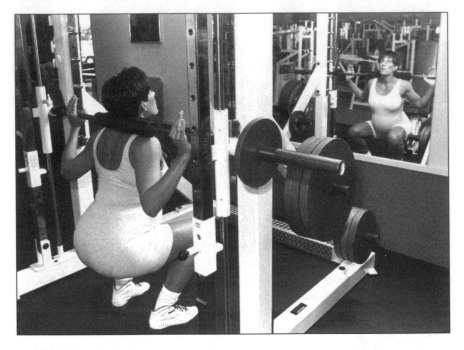

Figure 8.1   Weight training is OK in late pregnancy.

boredom pave the way for frequently missed workouts and guilt. Diversity also helps maintain interest.

The competitive athlete needs more focus and a regimen built around the needs of her specific sport. Strength training is usually an integral part of the regimen for these women (see figure 8.1) and appears to be an essential component for women who wish to improve their upper body strength.

Exercise Frequency, Duration, and Intensity

The effects of various training regimens on different aspects of fitness and physiological function suggest that the frequency, duration, and intensity of the exercise influence its ability to enhance the physiological adaptations to pregnancy. For example, the duration of moderate- to high-intensity exercise is an important determining factor of its cardiovascular effects. Over short and intermediate periods, cardiovascular function is well maintained. However, the volume changes associated with prolonged moderate- to high-intensity exercise can compromise cardiovascular function in the latter portion of a prolonged session.

Intensity is also important. For example, in young, healthy men sustained, low-intensity running, four or more times each week for a year does have a training effect on insulin response but does not alter body weight or increase maximal aerobic capacity. The same duration of exercise at a higher intensity has robust effects on body composition and maximal aerobic capacity (Oshida et al. 1989) and the same appears to be true during pregnancy.

Thus, it is likely that all these exercise performance variables have specific ranges during pregnancy that maximize the beneficial effects of exercise, like they do in the nonpregnant state. For example, think about the things that influence the baby's heart rate response to maternal exercise. It's clear that the greater the duration and intensity of the exercise, the greater the fetal heart rate response and probably the greater the reduction in uterine blood flow and blood glucose (Clapp, Little, and Capeless 1993). This means that the frequency, duration, and intensity of an exercise regimen will influence the 24-hour delivery of nutrients to the baby, which has a major influence on the baby's rate of growth. Therefore, with rigorous training regimens, the fetal heart rate and blood glucose responses to the training sessions are helpful guides in balancing the frequency, duration, and intensity of the workouts with the demands of the pregnancy. That is why I recommend that women who follow such a regimen involve a professional and consider volunteering as research subjects.

In addition, calculating the caloric demands of a specific exercise program and recording the timing of food intake helps in several ways. First, it helps a woman improve the quality and mix of the food she eats while ensuring adequate but not excessive caloric intake. For example, a common contributor to excessive weight gain is a decrease in exercise performance without an appropriate decrease in caloric intake. Second, it helps a woman prevent too little nutrient reaching the baby in late pregnancy. This can occur in mid- to late pregnancy during frequent, prolonged overdistance workouts (long duration, low- to moderate-intensity workouts) if sufficient calories are not eaten during and immediately after the exercise.

Threshold, Ceiling, and Dose-Response Effects

Most if not all training responses have both a threshold and a ceiling, or maximal response. Below a certain level of exercise performance (the threshold), there is no detectable effect on the response being examined. Above a certain level of exercise performance (the ceiling), there is no further improvement in the response, and it is common for the response to diminish (overtraining effect). In addition, between the threshold and the ceiling, most responses exhibit a dose-response effect (the greater the training stimulus, the greater the effect). The information in chapters 3 through 7 indicates that this is also the case in pregnancy. Furthermore, it turns out that the threshold and ceiling levels of exercise performance are different for different effects (for example, placental growth and birth weight). Indeed, my bet is that many training programs during pregnancy have not shown any effects on multiple facets of pregnancy outcome because they have not reached the threshold level of exercise necessary to produce the effects. As discussed in a previous section, the programs probably improve several aspects of maternal fitness but have little or no beneficial effect on the course and outcome of the pregnancy.

Decreasing Exercise

For the woman, too much exercise is signaled by the appearance of symptoms characteristic of the overtraining syndrome. Among others, these include fatigue, pain, loss of motivation, susceptibility to injury and common infections, and lackluster performances. The overtraining syndrome is common, and the same rules for avoiding it or treating it should apply during pregnancy. There is no reason I know to believe that pregnancy is any different, with one probable exception. Now there is a baby as well as a mother-to-be! So you must watch out for symptoms of *fetal overtraining* as well.

Decrease exercise volume if symptoms of overtraining develop in either the woman or the baby.

A practical way to monitor for overtraining is to frequently check for evidence of chronic fatigue. If this symptom develops, then the sensible solution is to modify either the exercise program or other lifestyle variables that produce fatigue (overtime at work, lack of sleep, and so on). If aches and pains persist, then the problem may be inappropriate or worn-out equipment or too much exercise. If the exercise is no longer fun and adding variety doesn't help, then the overall exercise load is probably too great. If recurrent upper respiratory or other illnesses develop, there probably is an imbalance in the amount of time spent in exercise versus that spent in restful activity. If there is a decrease in performance associated with an increase in the perceived level of exertion, then overtraining is a problem and modification is necessary. Finally, pay attention to any change in the baby's response to exercise and consider modification if needed, because what isn't too much for the mother could possibly be too much for the baby.

How will the baby let the mother know exercise is too much? Mom will know (see chapter 7). Remember, unborn babies are smart when it comes to dealing with stress (Clapp 1994b). First, if the exercise is interfering with the baby's getting enough nutrients, over time he will slow his growth rate, which should be obvious to the mother and her health care provider. Second, if the baby perceives any given exercise session as particularly stressful, he will not move much after the exercise. A good rule of thumb in mid- and late pregnancy is that the baby should usually move two or three times within the first 30 minutes after the exercise session is over. Finally, if there are concerns about the baby, it's reassuring to occasionally have someone listen to the baby's heart rate response to the exercise. Remember, the baby is no different from you or me; his heart rate goes up with a normal amount of stress. Up to the 32nd week, a normal response is an increase of 5 to 25 beats per minute. After that, as much as 30 to 35 beats per minute is OK. However, if the stress is more severe, the heart rate will rise more than that. If it is very severe, it may fall to levels 20 to 60 beats per minute lower than it was before exercise started. If any of these things occur, then I recommend the following:

- A medical evaluation should be done, including a detailed ultrasound exam with assessment of fetal behavior.
- If no cause can be found, the intensity and duration of the exercise regimen should be decreased by 10 to 25 percent.
- Arrangements should be made to monitor the fetal heart rate response frequently before and after exercise on the new regimen.

Increasing Exercise

Again, the answer to whether or not to increase exercise is simple. The volume of exercise, which is the product of average intensity and the time spent exercising each week, is not enough if there is little or no improvement in the fitness goals the woman has set. Remember, however, that all the different responses to training do not have the same threshold. The exercise goals must be very clear and focused and the types and patterns of exercise must be carefully chosen to ensure that the exercise will stimulate the desired responses. For example, specific types of strength training maximize explosive power and the ability to accelerate quickly (plyometrics or stationary jumps with weights are good examples). Although they do a lot for explosive power in the lower extremities, they do little to improve maximal aerobic capacity, speed over a longer distance, coordination, and so on. Thus, a woman needs to identify the exact training responses she desires in order to determine exactly what she needs to do to attain them. Then, she should start an exercise training regimen that employs the appropriate type of exercise at the appropriate frequency, duration, and intensity to produce an effect in every area of interest and check its progress on an ongoing basis.

Guidelines for Developing an Exercise Program

Now for the guidelines to use in developing a holistic program for women in each phase of the reproductive process. First, I summarize the current sanctioned guidelines and their recommended application in practice (American College of Obstetricians and Gynecologists 1994; Artal 1996; Artal and Buckenmeyer 1995). Then, I detail a more liberal and practical approach, pointing out where the differences lie.

Traditionally Sanctioned Guidelines

The guidelines and recommendations currently sanctioned by the policy makers in American obstetrics and the American College of Obstetricians and Gynecologists (ACOG) are condensed in table 8.1. Although they promote the value of regular exercise during pregnancy, they focus on avoiding any possibility of risk. To accomplish the latter, they recommend that a woman curtail the type, intensity, and duration of exercise during pregnancy and in the immediate postpartum period. Later in the chapter, I challenge the necessity of this approach and discuss it using the information in part II of this book. I present this approach here to offer another option as to which approach to follow during the different phases of the reproductive process.

Liberal, Practical Approach

The information in part II provides evidence indicating that regular exercise of various types is tolerated well by women and their offspring throughout the reproductive process. Accordingly, I have used that

Table 8.1

Sanctioned Guidelines for Exercise During Pregnancy for Otherwise Healthy Women

- Regular, moderate intensity and duration exercise sessions are preferable.
- Recommended exercises include stretching, stationary cycling, swimming, and walking. Other types are either contraindicated or require modification.
- Avoid jerky, bouncy, and wide range of motion movements and exercises that involve straining, jumping, or sudden changes in direction.
- Don't exercise lying on the back after the fourth month.
- Five-minute periods of warm-up and cool-down stretching are recommended, but don't stretch to the point of maximal resistance.
- Women with sedentary lifestyles should begin with short-duration, low-intensity activity and increase gradually.
- Stop exercise when fatigued; stop and consult a physician if any unusual symptoms occur.
- Increase caloric intake to cover the demands of the exercise and take fluids liberally before, during, and after exercise.
- Avoid environments with excessive heat and humidity when you exercise.

information to develop an alternative holistic but practical approach to exercise during pregnancy. It stresses consistency, education, and safety while balancing and integrating the demands of the exercise regimen with the needs of the pregnancy and other aspects of life. An integral and practical part of this approach is that it builds confidence and reduces anxiety by monitoring the progress of both the exercise regimen and the pregnancy. A brief discussion of each of its components follows.

Consistency

Reproduction and physical activity are both normal parts of life, and I've shown you that they complement one another functionally. So why all the fuss? Although there are some specific dos and don'ts that apply, there is no logical reason to change your approach to exercise prescription because the woman is passing through a phase of the reproductive process.

However, both the health care practitioner and the woman must play by the rules, whether she's trying to get pregnant, pregnant, or recovering from giving birth. Some women are tempted to show off a bit when exercising and pregnant to make a point (for example, when the woman is visited by an ambivalent or disapproving mother-in-law who's worried about her next grandchild). Likewise, some athletic women who firmly believe that exercise during pregnancy is a good thing feel they must do more when they are pregnant than they did before to make their point. Although they mean well, no one should use pregnancy and lactation as an excuse to do more or to disregard the rules that she would follow carefully when not pregnant. That's courting disaster, pregnant or not.

Education

In medicine there are two old adages that emphasize the importance of the education of both the doctor and the patient in the treatment of disease. They are

"A little knowledge is a bad thing."
and
"Knowledge and regular participation go hand in hand."

As far as I'm concerned, these old sayings apply to all types of prescription, including designing an exercise program. Indeed, they underlie the concept of licensure and qualification for professionals and the concept of focused education for others interested in a specific area. Simply put, designing a safe and adequate exercise program for various phases of the reproductive process requires an understanding of the interactions between exercise and the changes that occur in the different phases of the reproductive process. The goal of an educational component is to ensure that all concerned (the health fitness professional and the woman) have adequate information to alleviate unnecessary concern. This facilitates communication between individuals immensely and improves participation in and compliance with the overall plan.

If you think about it, there is a lot of information that both should know and understand. The minimum topics they should address include the following:

1. The basis of the theoretical concerns about exercise and reproduction and why, within broad limits, the concerns aren't supported by real scientific findings.

2. The important facts about the process of reproduction. Surprisingly, one of the most frequently asked questions by women contemplating pregnancy is "When in my cycle can I get pregnant?"

3. The impact the exercise has on each phase of the reproductive process and how the phase will influence the body's responses to exercise. For example, too much stress in one's life may interfere with ovarian function and heart rate response to exercise will change dramatically in early pregnancy.

4. The fact that both physical training and reproduction are not cut-and-dried. Both require commitment and flexibility to achieve the desired effect in the shortest time. Each requires balance with the other and with other aspects of life.

5. The reasoning behind a few commonsense dos and don'ts. For example, pregnant or not, understanding why hydration is good for the body and dehydration is bad will improve the likelihood of including adequate hydration before, during, and after exercise as part of the safety component of the overall program.

Interactive Component

It's important that the woman be intimately involved in developing the exercise plan to be sure that it will fit both her lifestyle and the changing needs and goals that develop with advancing pregnancy. If this doesn't happen, satisfaction and contentment decline, and missed workouts and guilt become problems. Each woman has her own objectives for exercising during pregnancy; thus, a successful individualized program is always designed with this in mind. For example, most women exercise because it relaxes them and improves their appearance and quality of life. Competitive performance is usually not a goal. Likewise, five sessions a week may not fit everybody's lifestyle and twice a day is for only a few.

The overall exercise program must fit
an individual's *goals* and *lifestyle.*

The interactions between lifestyle, the exercise regimen, and reproduction usually change as the reproductive process moves from one phase to the next. For example, the side effects from the hormonal signaling in early pregnancy and the demands of a new baby often dictate a temporary change in a woman's lifestyle as well as her exercise regimen. These changes are quite normal and should be anticipated and planned for by all concerned (see also chapters 9 through 11).

Instruction and Safety

Health care providers cannot take physical ability for granted when working with a woman to design an exercise program; thus, specific instruction and observation are often helpful. Not everyone knows the basics about equipment, stretching, warming up and cooling down, and so on. Moreover, proper biomechanics during an activity are important and should be observed and taught as needed by a qualified instructor. Few beginners naturally do it right. In the beginning runner, for example, stride length, heel strike, and excessive vertical motion are common problems. Posture and balance are important when using weights or a variety of training equipment (stair climbers, rowing machines, cross-country ski machines, and the like). A little instruction can avoid potential problems, making the exercise program a lot more fun and rewarding.

Indeed, assuming that either a beginner or an experienced exerciser will know and recognize what is and is not safe is often false. Knowledge in this area varies with the type of exercise, the experience of the individual, and the phase of the reproductive process. Such things as exercise surface, thermal environment, hydration, time of day, relationship to meals, and so on can be important safety issues and therefore demand a bit of thought. Likewise, many beginners overdo at first (unfortunately this holds for some more experienced exercisers as well). When someone is just beginning an exercise regimen, the premise that if a little is good then a lot will be better leads only to pain, injury, and the overtraining syndrome. A woman should understand and practice the concepts of rest-activity cycles and exercise as relaxation from the very beginning. Two good rules of thumb are an hour of restful activity for each hour of working out, and the amount of exercise that relaxes is good, but the amount that produces noticeable stress (muscle soreness, joint stiffness, cramping, fatigue, and the like) may be bad.

Monitoring

The health care provider and the woman should monitor both the exercise and the reproductive process. The detail required varies with the regimen and the reproductive phase: A serious training regimen requires using special monitoring techniques, whereas a not-so-serious regimen requires less. Table 8.2 shows a copy of the log we use to monitor exercise in our studies.

Additional nonexercise parameters to monitor include the following:

1. Feelings of well-being
2. Hydration
3. Weight
4. Nutrition
5. Rest-activity cycling

Which reproductive parameters should be monitored depends on the specific phase of pregnancy; see chapters 9 through 11.

If a problem arises with training, a fitness professional should evaluate it and work with the woman to take corrective action. Likewise, if any phase of the reproductive process is not proceeding normally, the woman and her health care provider should work together to handle it exactly like any other training problem: by thoroughly evaluating and treating it. If the evaluation indicates that the exercise regimen is contributing to the problem, the woman will have to modify or interrupt it for a time.

Comparing the Traditional and Liberal Approaches

There appears to be little if any need for restrictions during the time a woman is attempting pregnancy or following several months after the birth. However, during pregnancy and for the first two months after the birth, there are two schools of thought.

The first is conservative and suggests that stationary cycling and swimming are the best and safest types of exercise for both the mother and baby because they offer support for the mother and do not require balance or risk abdominal contact with another individual, ball, or other piece of equipment. Although masters-level swimmers and triathletes often maintain their competitive swimming skills during pregnancy (see figure 8.2), the learning curve for swimming, the requirement for specialized facilities (pool) and equipment (stationary bike), and the lack of diversity make this approach far from ideal for many women. Nonetheless, this specific recommendation is an important part of the current sanctioned guidelines (see table 8.1).

The second school of thought is based on the premise that if the woman takes appropriate safety precautions, the risk of injury is minimal for most types of exercise that are usually part of an exercise program. Therefore, the types of exercise are much more varied. In my opinion, this approach is more practical and realistic because it can

Table 8.2

Exercise Log

Name: _____ Log# _____

Date	Exercise type	Exercise duration	Average heart rate	RPE*	Comments

*Borg's Rating of Perceived Exertion:** 6–no exertion at all; 8–extremely light; 11–light; 13–somewhat hard; 15–hard (heavy); 17–very hard; 19–extremely hard; 20–maximal exertion.

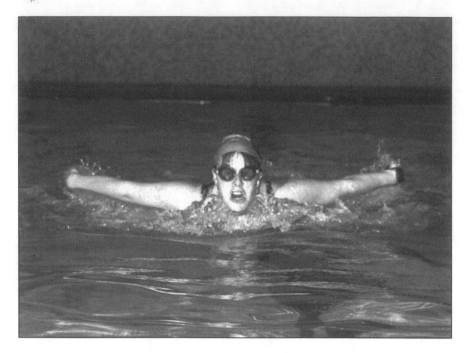

Figure 8.2   Swim training is OK in late pregnancy.

meet the fitness and lifestyle needs of most women without an appreciable increase in risk.

Although the current sanctioned guidelines (see table 8.1) discourage or prohibit many forms of exercise, exercise programs must be individualized. There are four principle factors to consider:

1. What phase of the reproductive process is the woman in? For example, unless she is more than 16 weeks pregnant, the risk of abdominal bumps and bruises harming the pregnancy is slim. So activities that involve contact or the risk of projectile trauma (hockey, softball, horseback riding, and the like) should be fine during the conception period, early pregnancy, and after the birth. Likewise, the repetitive sudden changes in vertical acceleration and deceleration in a variety of track and field endurance exercises might produce extreme breast discomfort during late pregnancy and lactation but are fine at other times.

2. What is the potential for injury? Certainly rock climbing without rope and harness or mountain bike racing carry greater risks of injury than ice or in-line skating.

3. How experienced is the individual?
4. What are her goals?

Use the answers to these four questions to jointly discuss and decide where to draw the line for risk versus benefit. I suggest that if either the pregnant woman or the health fitness professional is uncertain about the facts or uncomfortable with where to draw the line, seek additional professional advice. That's particularly important if there is any hint that the woman may have underlying disease. I touch on this in more detail in the following chapters.

To the best of my knowledge, there are no specific reports that document an increased incidence of injury during any phase of the reproductive process. As there are numerous reports documenting specific risk during other phases of life (childhood and adolescence for example), this suggests that the reproductive process itself is not a contraindication to many forms of exercise. The information currently available supports this view.

To date we have followed many women runners and women who have regularly performed one or more types of aerobics. We also have followed some women triathletes and women who cross-county ski, bike, swim, weight train, or use a stair climbing machine, rowing equipment, and the like. We have limited experience with racquet and ball sports, climbing, horseback riding, downhill skiing, water running, and contact sports. We are developing an in-depth experience with uphill treadmill walking. Others have had considerable experience with water aerobics, cycle ergometry, swimming, and circuit training. Maternal injuries of any type have been rare and fetal injury has not been recognized in any of these activities.

This lack of injury, however, is at least partly because most serious female athletes are practical, do worry about the possibility of injury, and voluntarily alter their approach. For example, both of the hockey players in our study stopped playing hockey by the 12th week of pregnancy but maintained a vigorous endurance-training program throughout. Racquetball players spontaneously decrease the sudden lateral motions required to return wall shots in late pregnancy, and downhill skiers ski with more emphasis on control and less on speed throughout mid- and late pregnancy. Runners continue to run, but they are much more particular about their shoes and the running surface. Serious weight trainers approach this activity with appropriate caution and help. But swimmers continue their racing starts and flip turns, and aerobics instructors, their power moves and step programs without apparent difficulty.

Dos and Don'ts

If a health care provider (or health fitness instructor) and the woman follow two basic rules, a prescribed exercise program can be safe and enjoyable throughout the reproductive process. First, always use common sense about what your body can do. Second, remember that the same general principles apply to exercise at all times. The list of dos and don'ts that follows illustrates how easy it is to develop an individualized program while following these two rules.

Dos

✓ *Approach the exercise program with breadth.* Focus on things other than performance, such as developing an improved sense of well-being, physical capacity, and productivity.

✓ *Make the exercise program fun and maybe even a little exciting.* It should be something to look forward to, not drudgery.

✓ *Make sure that the total volume of exercise is enough to enhance one's sense of well-being.* Anyone who has developed her own exercise program knows that until you reach a certain volume of exercise in a session, the rewards simply aren't there. For me it's 3.5 miles of running. For others it's 2, and for some it's between 5 and 10. Everyone is different, but it appears that 20 minutes at a moderately hard to hard level of perceived exertion is the minimum for most healthy women of reproductive age.

✓ *If it feels good, it's probably OK.* Whenever there is uncertainty, this is a practical rule to follow. This rule is particularly useful in late pregnancy for women who exercise with enthusiasm and lots of ballistic motion. Figure 8.3 makes this point. Note that abdominal support keeps the woman comfortable even while jumping during a vigorous step-aerobics routine.

✓ *Always chart progress and review it periodically.* This should provide a progressive sense of achievement. If it's not there, then there is something wrong with some part of the program.

✓ *Pay attention to the little things.* Hydration, rest-activity cycles, nutrition, and prompt attention to discomfort of any kind are as important as the exercise itself.

✓ *Pay as much attention to the reproductive process as you do to the exercise.* If the exercise is going well but the reproduction isn't, you have a problem that requires attention.

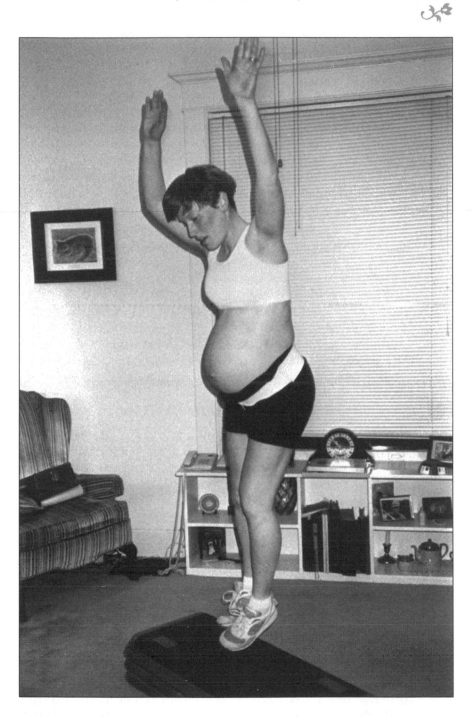

Figure 8.3   Ballistic motion and abdominal support in late pregnancy.

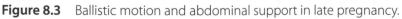

Don'ts

Most of the don'ts are the opposite of the dos. However, there are a few others that we should specifically mention.

✓ *Don't do something new without thinking it through.* This helps avoid doing things that can produce unpleasant or potentially harmful surprises. Two good examples of this involve travel. Before anyone travels from cool to hot or from sea level to high altitude, she should think about how the change in environment (temperature and oxygen tension) will influence her exercise capacity and her feelings of well-being (Pivarnik et al. 1992). I had a good friend who went to a meeting in Arizona where she went for her usual midday run on a beautiful desert road without a water bottle. About 30 minutes into the run, she started to feel dizzy, and, by the time she got back, she was badly dehydrated and her rectal temperature was 104 degrees. Not a smart thing to do, especially in very early pregnancy. Likewise, many women who live in the East or Midwest take off for an early ski weekend in Colorado or Utah on the spur of the moment. Unfortunately, however, many resorts are at 10,000 feet, and the top of the mountain is usually about 1,000 feet higher. If they are pregnant and not acclimated to this altitude, they often get so short of breath they have trouble sleeping, let alone skiing.

✓ *Don't be unprepared.* Never get into a new situation without advance preparation. A plan should always be in place to deal with injury, a sudden change in the environment, or sudden bleeding. This is particularly true for backcountry sports (hiking, climbing, mountain biking, ski touring, and the like), pregnant or not.

✓ *Don't continue if exercise produces pain.* If it hurts stop and evaluate. Pain with exercise is rarely a good sign and usually gets worse rather than better as time goes on. Particular attention should be paid to abdominal or pelvic pain, which may be the first sign of one of many problems that can occur throughout the reproductive process.

✓ *Don't ignore fatigue.* This is a difficult area to know where to draw the line. On the one hand, everyone gets tired. On the other, extreme, recurrent fatigue from physical stress in the workplace is the one symptom that is strongly associated with poor reproductive outcome in physically stressed working

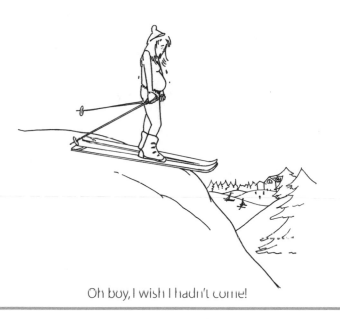

Oh boy, I wish I hadn't come!

women (Clapp 1996c; Luke et al. 1995; Mamelle, Laumon, and Lazar 1984).

How do you tell how much tiredness is normal and how much is too much? I use two guidelines here. First, if a woman is having difficulty getting other things done during the day because she is tired all the time or if she is dragging at the end of the day, that's too much until proven otherwise. Second, if the feelings of fatigue are accompanied by a noticeable decrease in motivation or performance, it's probably too much. Remember, however, that these responses may be the result of other life stress and not the exercise. Indeed, this often is the case in early pregnancy and immediately after giving birth. Because it can be hard to tell what the culprit is, I usually suggest that the woman either stop completely or cut way back on her exercise for a day or two to see what happens. If she feels better, she's been doing too much and should decrease her exercise load by 10 to 15 percent. However, often she feels worse because her personal time exercising was counteracting feelings of stress and fatigue rather than causing it. Under these circumstances, I encourage her to continue the exercise and look for a way to make other adjustments in her life, which usually resolves the problem.

✓ *Don't be rigid in the design of an individualized exercise program.* Be prepared to substitute one environment or activity for another or shift goals a little bit. For example, it may be wise to move inside to improve footing in the winter in the North or to avoid excessive heat stress in the summer in the South, even though the workout may have to be modified.

Contraindications to Exercise

In my view, save for a few notable exceptions, the contraindications to exercise for a healthy woman should be no different during the reproductive process than they are during other times in her life. Pregnancy is a normal physiologic state, not a disease, and the benefits of exercise appear to be substantial for both the woman and the pregnancy. Therefore, I believe that a healthy woman should be able to continue her exercise regimen while she is attempting to conceive and throughout early pregnancy without specifically seeking medical advice *unless* she develops one of the problems I discuss in this section.

The big four contraindications to exercise—
injury, disease, pain, bleeding.

Pregnant or not, there are four contraindications that usually require careful evaluation and therapy before beginning or resuming exercise. The first is straightforward—significant physical injury. The second is an acute bout of illness or chronic underlying disease, which is usually straightforward as well. Occasionally, however, difficult issues concerning immune function and prolonged recovery (especially recovery from respiratory illness and reconstructive surgery) can arise. In these situations, it is probably best to take a conservative approach, even for a highly motivated athlete. The third is the onset of persistent or recurrent localized pain. This always requires evaluation. The fourth is abnormal or heavy vaginal bleeding. Although this often turns out to be unrelated to the exercise, it is a warning sign that should not be ignored as it often is the first sign of previously unrecognized disease. There are a few additional contraindications, but they are limited to specific phases of the reproductive process. I address each in detail at the appropriate point in one of the next three chapters.

A more conservative approach is recommended in the current ACOG guidelines (1994). They put forth a series of absolute contraindications to exercise for healthy women. These have been broadly interpreted and expanded in the recent clinical literature to include relative contraindications (Artal 1996; Artal and Buckenmeyer 1995). A composite synopsis of these recommendations appears in table 8.3. Many of them are simply common sense and fall under my category of acute illness. However, objective evidence to support many others is lacking (multiple-birth pregnancy, history of premature labor, multiple miscarriages, and so forth), suggesting they may be unduly restrictive.

Table 8.3

Sanctioned Contraindications to Exercise During Pregnancy for Otherwise Healthy Women

Absolute contraindications	Relative contraindications
Pregnancy-induced hypertension	History of poor fetal growth
Ruptured membranes	History of rapid labors
Premature labor	Early pregnancy bleeding
Persistent bleeding after 12 weeks	Extreme overweight
A cervix that dilates ahead of schedule (incompetent cervix)	Extreme underweight
Poor fetal growth	Sedentary lifestyle
Multiple-birth pregnancy	Breech presentation after 28 weeks
Placental disease	Palpitations or arrhythmia
A history of three or more miscarriages or a history of premature labor	Anemia

Summary

The approach to exercise prescription for healthy women during the reproductive process should follow the same principles and use the same tools as those used at other times during life. I recommend a holistic approach that educates the woman and integrates and balances the exercise with the reproductive process and other aspects of life. Neither exercise nor reproduction exists in a vacuum, and both should be monitored serially to assess progress. Most healthy women with normal pregnancies do not require specific exercise prescription. However, women at the extremes of performance (beginners and serious athletes) as well as those who wish to increase their exercise regimen and improve fitness and performance during pregnancy will benefit from a detailed exercise prescription. The same is true for the woman with specific medical problems and needs. The right type, intensity, and frequency of exercise throughout the reproductive process are a function of the woman's fitness at the start and the goals she wishes to achieve. She may, however, need to cut back the exercise regimen if evidence of overtraining appears or an acute medical problem develops. But she may need to increase her regimen if she makes inadequate progress. In any case, three good rules to follow are an hour's restful activity for each hour's workout, the amount of exercise that relaxes is good but the amount that produces noticeable stress is bad, and when in doubt use common sense. In my view, the contraindications to exercise during the reproductive process are no different from other times during life. This approach differs from the one currently sanctioned by the medical community at large, which espouses conservative guidelines and contraindications.

CHAPTER 9

Preconception and Early Pregnancy

Although the physiological interactions are different, I've combined my comments about exercise prescription and monitoring for the preconception and early pregnancy phases of the reproductive process because they represent a continuum that is difficult to separate in a practical way. The fact of the matter is that early pregnancy is at least half over before a woman can be sure she is carrying a viable pregnancy.

I believe in emphasizing basic points and how they apply in different situations. So, I begin by reviewing what is known about the effects of exercise on three things that must happen properly to ensure normal conception. Next, I jog your memory about the importance of what is going on physiologically during these two phases, then I get to the specifics. As you'll see, although conception and early pregnancy have several specific problems, a major thrust of the exercise prescription during these phases is preparing the body for what it will need and benefit from later in the pregnancy.

Four Elements for Successful Conception

To become pregnant, a woman must produce a healthy egg, the womb must be ready to receive it, and the egg must be exposed to healthy sperm, all at the right time. If any of these factors does not exist, then pregnancy does not occur.

Four musts for conception—a healthy egg, a healthy sperm, a prepared womb, and timing.

Several systems in a woman's body must interact with one another in a precise way to mature and release a viable egg from an ovary (figure 9.1). Signals from the hypothalamus in her brain stimulate her pituitary gland to release periodic pulses of protein hormones. These hormones then stimulate the ovarian tissues to mature and release the egg. It's more complicated, however, because they also stimulate the ovaries to release hormones of their own (estrogen and progesterone), which do two things. First, they circulate back to the pituitary gland and hypothalamus and fine-tune the timing of their stimulatory activity. This keeps the process of egg maturation and release on an exact schedule. Second, they prepare the lining of the womb so it is ready to receive and support a fertilized egg.

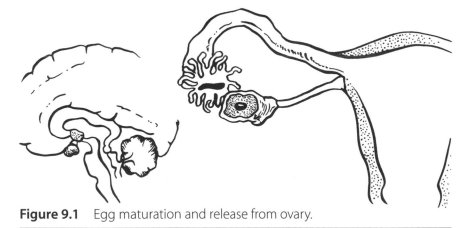

Figure 9.1   Egg maturation and release from ovary.

A similar process is involved in producing sperm in a man's testicles. The only differences are that the process is continuous rather than cyclic, and the process of sperm production through maturation takes longer from start to finish (six to eight weeks). Then, intercourse must occur near the time the ovary releases the egg so viable sperm will be present in the woman's fallopian tube to fertilize the egg shortly after it's released. Finally, the fertilized egg must travel to the uterus and arrive at the right time to implant.

Obviously, it's a complicated system, but if the timing is right, it works with no apparent problem 90 to 95 percent of the time. So why worry about a little exercise? Well, it appears that exercise training can contribute to problems with the system's function in four well defined ways.

1. When a woman's brain senses that she is under a lot of stress (mental, physical, or nutritional), it signals the hypothalamus that it's not a good time to get pregnant, and the hypothalamus stops sending signals to the pituitary gland. In turn, the pituitary stops sending signals to the ovaries, the ovaries stop releasing eggs and hormones, and menstrual periods stop. When the stress decreases the brain says, "Hey, now it's OK," and the system starts again.

This is a normal protective response and happens frequently to women under stressful circumstances (going away to college, dieting, new job, death in the family, moving to a new area, chronic disease, and so on). The level of stress required to cause it is highly variable from woman to woman. When exercise training gets to a level that creates physical, mental, and nutritional stress, the body acts the same way. Thus, it's not unusual for a competitive athlete to experience this when she's peaking for her competitive season, but it usually goes away for the rest of the year. It also occurs in women who do a lot less exercise but have a variety of other stressors in their lives (work, relationships, eating disorder, and so on). The question often comes down to whether it is the exercise or the stress. My experience says, most of the time, it is the other stressors, not the exercise.

2. There is some convincing evidence (Loucks 1996; Loucks et al. 1992) that the same thing can happen in a subtle way in women athletes who develop a minor energy imbalance (caloric intake versus energy expenditure). In these cases, menstrual periods remain normal, but there appears to be a disruption in thyroid function. It alters the frequency of pulsatile release of one or more of the protein hormones from the pituitary gland. A change in the pattern of these sudden increases and decreases in hormonal levels can disrupt ovarian release of

estrogen and other hormones. This may interfere with ovulation and the receptivity of the lining of the womb and usually shortens cycle length as well (called a luteal phase defect). Although the direct effect of this on fertility has yet to be examined in an exercise populace, any one of these could potentially impair a woman's ability to conceive.

3. One symptom of overtraining and fatigue is a decline in sexual interest and activity. Remember, it takes more than a lonesome egg in the fallopian tube to become pregnant!

4. When conception is difficult, it's often because the man does not produce an adequate number of viable sperm. Although the effect of exercise on sperm production is not well studied, it is clear that a stress syndrome similar to that described in women occurs in some male athletes and is associated with low sperm counts and loss of sexual interest (Ayers et al. 1985; Eichner 1992). In addition, sperm viability is dramatically decreased by small increases in the temperature of the testicles. There is good reason to believe that this may be happening during training when athletes wear tight-fitting synthetic fabrics for protracted periods (triathlete gear is a prime example). Although this has not been studied in humans, it may play a role in the isolated cases of unexplained low sperm counts found in male endurance athletes. Interestingly, one of the first methods of contraception was to have the male take a prolonged bath in hot water nightly to decrease his fertility by killing sperm. The same effect could easily be happening during a prolonged training session on a hot day. At any rate, the effect of exercise gear on testicular temperature during endurance training deserves more attention.

Physiological Function Before Conception

Although a woman's physiological function is unchanged during the preconceptional phase, she should place physiological emphasis on making sure that all systems are *go* before she attempts pregnancy. This helps ensure that the initial interaction between the exercise and the reproductive process will go smoothly.

Trying to get pregnant definitely is not the time to be peaking for major competition and, ideally, the woman's exercise regimen should be at a plateau. She should also be as healthy as possible. In addition to the usual attributes of health, this means being well nourished, ovulating regularly, and being mentally prepared for the changes that early pregnancy brings. If any of these areas require attention, now is the time to address it, because a problem in any of them increases the chance of more problems later. For example, the activity and magnitude of any underlying disease and what its impact will be during pregnancy are much easier to assess before conception has occurred. Likewise, if there are problems with either the amount or mix of nutrients, now is the time to change it because the symptoms of early pregnancy often interfere once conception has occurred.

As you well know, a woman must ovulate to get pregnant. So, if there are questions or concerns in this area and there is a rush to become pregnant (age or other commitment), a woman's ovulatory status should be checked out before trying to conceive, rather than one year after beginning to try to conceive. Now is the time for a woman to learn about early pregnancy so the changes her body encounters will not be a surprise. It usually is difficult for anyone to alter her lifestyle significantly in a short time, and, once pregnant, time is very, very short!

Physiological Function in Early Pregnancy

Early pregnancy encompasses the first 8 weeks after conception or about the first 10 weeks after the first day of the last menstrual period. Physiologically, this is a time of rapid and sometimes tumultuous change for both the baby and mother-to-be. This is when the baby develops in only a few days from one cell into a ball of cells, which then rapidly become different tissues. These tissues grow and differentiate to form all the organs and organ systems that serve the baby for the remainder of its life. Naturally, it's really important that everything goes well.

At the same time, the hormonal signals from the baby and its placenta reset how the mother's organ systems respond to many things, and the mother usually doesn't feel well while this readjustment is occurring. Many of her body's responses to exercise change over this time interval. Most women will suffer all the symptoms of *underfill*: their heart rates will be high, and they may feel dizzy, especially right after exercise. Most will feel hot, tired, and short of breath all the time. Their noses will probably be stuffy, they may suffer from an upset stomach, and they'll never stray far from a bathroom.

Nonetheless, this is a point in pregnancy when the interactive effects of exercise stimulate the early growth of the placenta and its vasculature, enhance multiple facets of the maternal adaptations to pregnancy, and, in the process, usually improve many unpleasant symptoms of early pregnancy. Therefore, it's important for a woman to keep up the exercise if she wants to reap the benefits from the interaction. Long-term that's important because it is these early benefits that provide the margin of safety, allowing her to do more later.

Contraindications to Exercise

First, I want emphasize that there are specific symptoms during these two phases that require evaluation before beginning or continuing exercise for all women. They include the following:

- Absent or infrequent menstrual periods
- Injury
- Acute illness
- Vaginal bleeding with or without cramping in early pregnancy
- Intractable nausea and vomiting
- Sudden onset of new pain, especially in the abdomen or pelvis

These are all signs of significant problems, and, depending on the findings, it may be necessary to either modify or stop exercise for a time.

Now to the details of exercise prescription for three groups of women from the time they attempt pregnancy until they are 10 weeks beyond the start of their last menstrual period. Keep in mind that even after studying this material, when in doubt, common sense and consistency are the way to go.

Beginning Exercisers

Making a long-term lifestyle change, like starting an exercise regimen, only succeeds if the individual consistently follows an exercise program and obtains meaningful rewards for doing so. This is even more important for an individual who has tried but failed in the past. The other rule for beginners is don't do too much too fast.

Education

Knowing the positive effects of exercise on pregnancy and alleviating any concerns makes it easier for an individual to stick to a regimen. Important points that every woman and health fitness professional working with her should know include the following:

- The basics of menstrual rhythms and function, conception, and early pregnancy

- The effects of exercise on the menstrual cycle, ovulation, and early pregnancy
- The effects of pregnancy on the body's response to exercise

Clinician's Guide for Educating Beginning Exercisers About Pregnancy

To do it right, plan at least two or three educational sessions. Most people can only digest and retain four or five points in a session, and there is a lot of information to cover. You may want to develop your own highlighted handout for each session and give each woman a copy. This maintains attention during the session, and participants can use it as a reference later on. Keep it simple and do not cover too much too fast. Begin with the basics and build on them.

- Cover the basics of menstrual rhythms, conception, and early pregnancy.
- Define the ranges of normal menstrual function (25 to 35 days in length, 2 to 6 days of flow, starts heavy, gets light, and so on).
- Point out common abnormalities (spotting, occasional missed periods, effect of stress or illness, and so on).
- Discuss the time in the cycle when a woman is likely to be fertile (12 to 17 days before her next expected period, although recent evidence suggests that it can go to 19 days in some women).
- Mention several ways to determine if ovulation is occurring regularly (rise in rectal temperature, sudden clear, copious vaginal discharge, and so on).
- Discuss the changes and symptoms of early pregnancy and point out that, during this time interval, there is a rapid formation of new embryonic tissues that will ultimately become the baby.

After this background, cover the effects of exercise on the menstrual cycle, ovulation, and the functional changes that occur in a woman's body during early pregnancy. Point out how these changes affect her body's response to exercise. Be sure to specify issues that bear directly on individual decisions (disruption in ovarian function and menstrual cyclicity, weight gain, fat accretion, blood volume expansion, heart rate during exercise, blood sugar responses to exercise, the increased sensation of shortness of breath, feelings of dizziness and warmth, and so on). Then make it clear that two new things (exercise and pregnancy) at the same time occasionally interfere with one another (use ovulation as an

cont'd ☞

example). Use that logic to explain why you recommend she follow one of two initial plans.

Ideally, she should begin the exercise regimen six weeks or more before she gets pregnant so her body is used to the exercise before it has to deal with the pregnancy. But if she can't wait or is already pregnant, she should begin at a level that involves no more than three 20-minute sessions a week, at a moderate level of perceived exertion and keep it there until early pregnancy is over.

End by giving the woman the opportunity to ask questions or discuss points that apply specifically to her situation. If she has questions you can't answer, find the answers or send her to see someone who can.

Interactive Component

Making sure that the exercise regimen is fun and fits one's lifestyle like a glove maximizes both faithful participation in the program and reward from it. This is especially important for a woman who is beginning an exercise program, and the woman and her health fitness provider must spend some time talking about her overall life in order to develop a program that works. It is really helpful if there are clear answers to the following questions:

- What types of exercise are enjoyable?
- How much free time is available for exercise?
- What time of day is free?
- What types of facilities are available?
- Is there a gym or an outdoor track accessible?
- Do any friends or members of her family have exercise equipment at home?
- Is there anyone available to exercise with?
- Are there other commitments (childcare, career, running a household, committee work, and so on) to work around?
- Can she or others do anything to make more time for exercise if needed?

Using a few additional planning tricks makes the exercise program more fun and can really motivate a woman to continue exercising long-term. These won't work, however, unless they mesh well with a woman's lifestyle habits and goals. This is why the basic information is necessary. The planning tricks include the following:

✓ *Start the day with exercise.* I recommend starting the day with exercise because the first goal in one's day almost always gets accomplished. Things frequently arise in everyone's day that require a change in plan, and, if an individual has already done the exercise, then it's not the thing she puts aside to solve the time bind. Most beginners indicate that they feel better after exercise. So if a woman exercises early in the day, it usually makes the next few hours easier and more productive, which provides positive reinforcement to continue.

✓ *Exercise with a friend or group.* Exercising in a social setting either with a friend or a group inevitably makes it more fun, assures greater compliance with the regimen, and provides positive feedback. Togetherness exerts a subtle pressure to conform because with it comes an exercise commitment to someone other than oneself. Likewise, if an individual's motivation is low on any day, the fact that she'll have the opportunity to finish yesterday's conversation or see someone she otherwise would not see usually provides incentive. These are some of the reasons that aerobics are so popular, and, for many women in this category, it's a good choice if it's affordable and fits.

✓ *Build rewards into the prescription.* I try to tailor rewards to the obvious likes and dislikes of an individual woman and often include them in more than one part of the prescription. You can make them part of the rest-activity cycling (massage, movie, and so on), the nutritional component (a favorite but "naughty" snack), the safety component (new shoes or outfit every X number of sessions), or the evaluation component (physical appearance, waist size, skinfold thickness, strength, endurance, and so on).

✓ *Keep an exercise log and diary to encourage a feeling of accomplishment.* It can be used by both the exercising woman and her health fitness practitioner to look back and see how much better she feels now than she did when first starting exercise.

✓ *Avoid anything other than transitory discomfort or inconvenience until the regimen is fully integrated into everyday life.* The rule of thumb I use to determine when the transitory discomfort is gone is when the woman spontaneously starts showing her health care provider the exercise logs and asks about increasing the exercise load. Although this means that the health care provider may have to accept a slower start than desired, you often both get where you want to go sooner than you would otherwise.

✓   *Keep in mind that ultimately the exerciser should always make the final decision to alter the exercise regimen.* Health fitness instructors or health care providers may suggest and prod when they feel the time is right, but ultimately the decision must be the woman's if it's going to work. For example, if the fatigue and nausea of early pregnancy make a woman want to temporarily back off or modify the regimen, no one should discourage her from doing so. Remember, these symptoms indicate the pregnancy is normal and the symptoms are often relieved by short (three- to five-minute) bouts of activity when they are at their worst.

Type of Exercise

The next step is to decide what type of exercise will be adequate to achieve the objectives the two of you have agreed on. Usually this includes some combination of fun, fitness, weight control, appearance, strength, preventive health, specific skill development, and well-being. In this group, competitive performance is rarely if ever included.

I'm a believer in a three-pronged approach to exercise prescription for women who are beginning to exercise. I recommend combining a weight-bearing exercise that the woman likes and can continue for a minimum of 20 minutes (running, uphill treadmill walking, aerobics, or stair climbing) with stretching exercises and strength training. I like this approach because it improves endurance, flexibility, and strength all at once and usually has a rapid, noticeable effect on body configuration, function, and sense of well-being. In addition, as the motions often mimic those we use daily, its effects on an individual's physical performance in everyday life are often striking. Most aerobics classes include all these components and therefore are good choices, but only if they fit the woman's lifestyle. If the expense or the schedules of health clubs, YWCAs or YMCAs, or the like don't fit and she likes the regimen, there are videotapes or cable exercise programs to fall back on.

There are, however, many alternatives. If the woman must fit exercise in whenever she can, then it needs to be independent of fitness facilities or at least group programs. For this individual, combining a stretching, resistance-band regimen with brisk walking that evolves into walk-jog, then jogging, often works well.

A variety of circuit-training regimens produce excellent effects, but they have limited accessibility and require a variety of skills. Several machines available at fitness facilities work well. These include a variety of step and cross-country ski machines. They can also be purchased ($300 to $1,000 new, much less if purchased used) for home use. Their drawbacks are that they have a learning curve, and, like cycle ergometry, they rapidly become boring even when combined with another activity (reading, watching TV, socializing, or the like). Although not weight-bearing, swimming is another alternative, but without prior experience or coaching and preconditioning it's often tiring and frustrating because its skills are not acquired rapidly. In addition, many former swimmers find lap swimming boring. Most other activities that women find fun (racquet and ball sports, water sports, hockey, weight training, and so on) are intermittent activities that require either a preconditioning period or special skills. They should not usually be part of the initial exercise regimen for a woman starting regular exercise for the first time.

Exercise Instruction and Safety

Once the exercise regimen is in place, develop a list of the necessary clothing and equipment and where to buy them. Appropriate, quality footwear is especially important. Beginning a walk-jog regimen using an old pair of tennis shoes or lounging sneakers is a clear invitation to soreness and possibly injury as well.

The health fitness or health care provider should observe at least the 1st, 5th, and 10th exercise sessions to be sure that the woman's biomechanics are correct, the environment is safe, and the woman is having fun and progressing. After that the need for instruction is highly variable, individualized, and usually can be combined with monitoring.

The next safety issue is how much, how fast? My advice is to rely on the individual and her perceptions of how she feels and when she feels she is ready. It is important, however, to also remember that the exerciser must achieve a level of performance that exceeds the threshold necessary for the rewards. At a minimum, start with 20- to 30-minute sessions, three times a week, at a moderate level of perceived exertion. If the woman is in a rush to conceive or is newly pregnant, keep it at that level until early pregnancy is complete.

Avoid doing too much too fast.

If, however, you have time before conception, I recommend increasing some aspect of the performance every 6 to 10 sessions. This is slow enough to avoid injury and fast enough for the woman to experience noticeable progress. I usually start by increasing workload (cadence, range of motion, or speed) because it gives the individual a sense of progress. Then I increase the duration (five minutes at a time). The last thing I change is the frequency, because if frequency is changed too soon, the chances of discomfort or injury increase. After conception occurs or if conception does not occur in the ensuing three to four months, space out increases further to every 10 to 15 sessions.

Finally, there are several important things to consider about environmental conditions, eating patterns, rest-activity cycling, hydration, and so on that I cover in detail under the dos and don'ts.

Monitoring

In women beginning a regular exercise program, monitoring does not need to be intense. It should focus on evaluating progress and the physiological responses in both domains. In our experience, if pregnancy does not occur within three to six cycles in which there has been adequate sexual contact, then there is a problem with progress in the reproductive domain (usually unrelated to the exercise) that requires attention. At that point, I suggest that the woman contact her doctor for further evaluation. This is particularly true if the woman has had regular cycles with evidence of ovulation.

I also recommend that women keep a log of their menstrual cycles and sexual contacts on a calendar when attempting pregnancy because, exercise or not, keeping this history can save time later if they have difficulty conceiving. I have yet to see evidence that beginning the type of exercise regimen we outline interferes with the regularity of the menstrual cycle (indeed, it may improve it). However, my experience with this group of women is still limited, and it's a good idea to ask them to keep track.

In early pregnancy, I recommend that the woman monitor three things that indicate everything is progressing normally with the pregnancy, and I ask her to write them down periodically. How does she feel in terms of well-being (once a week)? How much weight has she gained (twice a month)? Is she depositing fat over her hips, thighs, and abdomen (twice a month)? Some normal responses to these respective questions would be "Not so good," "One and a half to two pounds plus," and "Yes, lots."

Monitoring the progress and responses to exercise in the precon- ceptional and early pregnancy phases overlaps a bit. How a woman feels (fatigue, well-being, and so on) is important in safeguarding against overtraining during these two phases and in deciding whether to modify the exercise (see chapter 3 for details). Progress in performance should be slow but steady and is perhaps best assessed by subjective changes in capacity, endurance, and satisfaction. The exercise-associated increases in heart rate will jump at the time of conception. Rather than judging exercise intensity via heart rate during these phases, a woman should measure intensity using the Borg Rating of Perceived Exertion scale (see figure 3.2, p. 53). Check the thermal response periodically for re- assurance and check weight loss with a typical session as an index of fluid depletion. Once every week or two is plenty. The best check of dietary adequacy is a stable weight before conception, followed by a gradual 6- to 10-pound weight gain over the ensuing eight weeks.

Dos and Don'ts

✓ *Pay attention to environmental conditions, especially thermal ones.* A woman should avoid significant hyperthermia when attempt- ing to get pregnant and throughout early pregnancy. The ther- mal adaptations to both regular exercise and pregnancy make it easy to do as long as the woman avoids exercising in a hot or humid environment. I discourage running at midday when the sun is out, exercising in gymnasiums without air-conditioning or with poor air circulation, and so forth. Most health care pro- fessionals also recommend staying away from hot tubs, saunas, and steam baths in early pregnancy. But our limited experience and that of others indicates that most pregnant women sponta- neously get out of the hot tub, sauna, or steam room long be- fore their core temperatures rise significantly. At this point in time the practical answer for the individual woman who enjoys one of these postexercise treats is to simply check her rectal or vaginal temperature several times when she gets out. If it is under 38 degrees centigrade (100.4 degrees Fahrenheit) then it probably is alright to continue.

✓ *Pay attention to hydration and salt intake.* Hydration is important to cardiovascular stability at all times, but especially in early pregnancy when the vascular underfill needs to be corrected (see chapter 2). The best way an individual can support hydra- tion is by maintaining salt intake and drinking enough all day and during exercise to keep the urine so dilute it's virtually clear (like water). Don't exercise when dehydrated and don't exercise without water are two practical rules that make the point. Morning exercisers should be sure to drink water when they get up to urinate at night.

✓ *Pay attention to eating patterns.* It appears best for the early development of the baby if mothers-to-be avoid having their blood sugar fall to low levels. Because of the metabolic changes going on this can be a real problem that requires attention. To avoid low blood sugar levels in early pregnancy, a woman needs to eat small quantities of specific types of carbohydrate (fruits, peas, beans, salads, pastas, nuts, whole grain breads, and ice cream) frequently (every three hours during the day plus a bedtime snack). The type of carbohydrate is very important; processed types of starches and potatoes (most cereals, white bread, donuts, french fries, chips, pretzels, popcorn, cakes, cookies and most other snack foods except ice cream) can actually cause the blood sugar to fall rapidly about one hour after eating, which is not good for the baby and also makes most women ravenously hungry so they end up eating more than they should. The best plan is to get the body used to this pattern of eating and this type of carbohydrate before pregnancy, because it also helps relieve the early pregnancy symptom of nausea. The timing of food intake relative to the exercise sessions is also important. Exercise sessions should not begin in the first two hours after eating and the woman should eat a small snack right after her exercise session. If she follows my advice and exercises first thing in the morning she should plan a liquid snack during the exercise with a small breakfast to follow. Fasting for more than four hours should be avoided and rapid weight gain should be viewed as quite normal in early pregnancy.

✓ *Avoid excessive fatigue.* At this time, a woman's body needs its rest, as well as its exercise, more than usual. Even if a woman is not trying to become pregnant, avoiding fatigue is so important to feeling and doing well that exercise specialists have coined a phrase for it—rest-activity cycling. In practical terms, this means at least an hour of quiet time fun for each hour of planned exercise. If this is a problem, take steps to decrease other time commitments. Right now the reproductive process and the exercise should be the woman's main priorities.

✓ *Confirm pregnancy as soon as possible after probable conception.* It is a good idea to confirm the fact that conception has occurred. These days that's easy enough to do. Pregnancy tests for home use are easy to perform, require only a few drops of urine, and are accurate, sensitive, and readily available. The result clarifies the situation for all concerned, and an early positive is very helpful in establishing the estimated date for delivery with greater certainty. Many women in this group also decide to see their doctor early for reassurance that everything is A-OK. If so, I recommend that the visit take place about eight weeks after their last menstrual period. Waiting until then ensures that an abdominal ultrasound examination can accurately confirm fetal viability and whether or not it is a multiple-birth pregnancy.

✓ *Stop and evaluate.* If localized pain, vaginal bleeding, or a sudden change in feelings of well-being occur, exercise should be stopped and the woman should be evaluated (preferably by the doctor or midwife she plans to see) to determine the cause.

The common sense approach says keep cool,
hydrated, well rested, and well fed.

Recreational Athletes

I call women who exercise regularly for fun and health recreational athletes because they rarely compete. They are some of the easiest individuals to design an exercise program for because they only want to do a bit more than they are currently doing and feel better than average during pregnancy. Their motivation and commitment is clear, and, for most, their goals are attainable. Usually, they are a curious group full of questions. For these women, explanation, encouragement, and monitoring for reassurance are all that is necessary.

Education

With this group, concern is usually not the issue. They already subscribe to the view that exercise is safe or they wouldn't be interested in expanding their exercise program during pregnancy. They exercise for fun and aren't particularly interested in competition. They're curious and want explanations and guidance in several areas. Here are several examples:

- Will more exercise improve feelings of well-being?
- Will it make the pregnancy, labor, and delivery easier?
- Exactly what should be done to get the most benefit?
- What usually happens to the level of exercise performance later in the pregnancy?
- Is exercise comfortable later in pregnancy?

Clinician's Guide for Educating Recreational Exercisers About Pregnancy

For this group, you should cover the same basic material in the first session (menstrual cycle, the changes and problems of early pregnancy, and so forth). Then focus on what they really want to know in the second session. Be prepared for many questions. A handout is a good idea for this group as well, and you should be prepared to recommend additional reading about both exercise and pregnancy.

I usually begin the second session by talking about how regular exercise training changes the way the body works and what will happen if they do more (threshold and dose-response effects). Then, I move on to how regular exercise improves the changes induced by pregnancy. Next, I present its benefits and end with a discussion of its potential risks during these early phases of the reproductive process. Throughout, I emphasize that a gradual increase in exercise performance coupled with appropriate monitoring will maximize benefit and minimize risk.

I find that's all it takes. Within that format their questions give you plenty of opportunity to discuss sexual activity, ovulation, nutrition, rest, temperature regulation, fluid replacement, and so on. At the end, when you ask them if they have any other questions, be prepared to spend another 10 to 20 minutes answering them. In addition, expect a call now and then to clear something up that has just occurred to someone.

Interactive Component

Most recreational athletes have little difficulty integrating gradual increases in exercise performance with becoming pregnant and the rest of their lives. Most have already developed a stable lifestyle with personal time built in and are more than willing to move other things around to make time for the monitoring and so on. They are ready to become a parent and recognize the need for flexibility and compromise if difficulties arise with either the exercise or the reproductive process. Trust, adherence to the fitness program, and teamwork among these women and both medical and fitness personnel are usually nonissues. In fact, if a difficulty does arise in these areas, the issue is usually rapidly resolved by a switch in providers.

Setting Goals

Most women in this group need to develop goals in only two areas. Skill, speed, and distance are only occasionally important, but demonstrable improved fitness and an improved sense of well-being during pregnancy always are. To accomplish the former, I recommend focusing on two or more aspects of fitness important to the individual (endurance, strength, flexibility, appearance, and so on). Then develop a plan that should improve these aspects, including a monitoring component that will demonstrate progress, pregnant or not. Unless there is a compelling reason, I recommend not developing goals in the areas of new skills, speed, and balance because progress in these areas may be difficult to demonstrate later in the pregnancy. The improved sense of well-being requires all concerned to pay strict attention to be sure that the rate of change in exercise load is balanced by an equivalent increase in quiet rest. Otherwise, symptoms of overtraining may appear. If the rest-activity cycles are balanced appropriately, then an individual's sense of well-being invariably increases with an increase in exercise volume and greater exercise diversity. It is easily demonstrated in two ways: by keeping a log and by comparing oneself with other women.

Type of Exercise

I also recommend a combined exercise program for the recreational athlete because I believe that many of their programs are too focused on one particular activity. Accordingly, design the new program to be more diverse, including endurance, strength, and flexibility components.

Endurance

I usually keep a woman's current endurance component but also introduce at least one alternate type of exercise in case she needs it later in the pregnancy. I base the alternative on the woman's physical configuration and exercise type. For example, relatively short women runners usually run out of room between their ribs and pelvic girdle in late pregnancy. As a result, the growing uterus has nowhere to go but out, the abdomen protrudes excessively, and the uterus and baby often rest on the anterior arch of the pelvis and move up and down with each stride. Although abdominal support usually helps, this can be quite uncomfortable and maintaining exercise intensity, frequency, and duration may require a change from running to stair stepping, low-impact aerobics, a cross-country ski machine, or water jogging. If a woman becomes familiar with one of the alternatives early on, transitioning to it in late pregnancy will be smooth and easy. The same holds true for many women whose primary focus is a racquet or ball sport, ice hockey, gymnastics, or the like. Most profit from a more defined yet varied endurance component that gradually supersedes their primary endeavor as pregnancy progresses.

I do recommend, however, limiting abrupt changes in the endurance component in either very early pregnancy or while a woman is attempting to become pregnant. The rationale for not doing more at this time is if it's working well now (ovulation, hormonal milieu of early pregnancy, thermoregulation, and so forth), don't tinker with it—or maybe it won't. Therefore, I limit increasing the time spent in endurance workouts to a total of an additional 30 minutes a week throughout these two phases.

Strength

I also recommend that recreational athletes either start or continue a weight-training program that focuses on improving upper body strength. This is something that many need, and it's easy to see rapid progress. If the woman already strength trains, I ask her to continue her current regimen and not to increase either her weight loads, repetitions, or sets until later in the pregnancy (10 to 12 weeks). For women who have never weight trained, I recommend beginning with light free weights and incorporating upper extremity motion with weights into the endurance part of her program. Aerobics is the ideal type of exercise for this, but a woman can incorporate it into running, stepping, and so on. The only problem is balance. So I don't recommend anything over three to four pounds until the woman is ready for machines or a separate free weight program. These can be introduced at any time throughout these two phases or before the 28th week of pregnancy. After that it's a bit difficult to start either. I usually include the transition as part of the plan but let the woman decide when she is ready to begin it.

Flexibility

Stretching should be a part of everyone's exercise program, pregnant or not. It maintains an individual's range of motion, avoids tightness, pain, and cramping, and may actually decrease the incidence of muscle injury. The problem is it takes time and most people are in a hurry, so many people often neglect it. So keep in mind that during pregnancy stretching also can do the following:

1. Help maintain normal posture and balance
2. Give a woman the assurance that she can continue to assume a wide range of postures and do things requiring a fair amount of extension
3. Improve a woman's sense of well-being and confidence

Flexibility is best maintained or improved by introducing a series of stretching exercises as part of the cool-down portion of the endurance component when the muscles are already warm and perhaps less susceptible to injury. There is no reason to exclude any stretching position including those performed on the back during these two phases, and, if flexibility and coordination are major goals, it's easy to expand this component of the exercise program over time.

While current guidelines recommend avoiding maximal extension during pregnancy, there is no objective evidence that it is harmful or increases the incidence of dislocation. The only unanswered question involves the safety of supine floor exercises in late pregnancy, an issue that is currently under study in my laboratory.

Again, a program of aerobics is the most efficient and fun way to combine these three components, but, as discussed earlier, there are many alternatives. It all depends on the woman, her preferences, and her lifestyle.

Instruction and Safety

Maintaining a program of regular recreational exercise does not automatically mean that the individual is using proper equipment or facilities and has correct biomechanics. Equipment should be checked to be sure it is in good condition; the workout environment should have stable, even surfaces; and the temperature should not be over 85 degrees Fahrenheit. This last point can be a difficult one in either the aerobics or weight rooms of many health clubs in the summer time, because it costs money to keep these areas cool. Check it if there is any question that a room is too warm, and if so see that it is changed. Biomechanical problems and instruction as to how to avoid them or how to change a workout require evaluation by a health fitness professional. This is a worthwhile investment for most recreational athletes, especially those preparing to deal with the changes in body configuration that accompany pregnancy.

My only other safety concern involves *being prepared* and *thinking before you act*. Usually this is not a problem because most of these women's exercise routines are well established. When a woman travels, however, she sometimes starts something she wishes she hadn't (skiing at altitude is the perfect example). Here common sense provides the best rule of thumb to follow: if it doesn't feel good, don't continue to do it!

Monitoring

Monitoring progress toward individual exercise goals is central for recreational athletes. Conception is rarely a problem in recreational athletes, so monitoring the reproductive process needs only a careful confirmation of the due date (need dates of the last menstrual period and date of an early pregnancy test that's positive) and documentation that weight gain is occurring at the normal rate. At this point, monitoring the responses to exercise is only cautionary and should focus on detecting changes in perceived exertion and the thermal response.

Both progress in performance and the physiological responses to the changes in the exercise regimen should be evaluated after two weeks. Thereafter, they should be evaluated monthly. If the progress in performance is slow, it may be necessary to increase one or more components of the training regimen, and if there is evidence of stress (pain, undue fatigue, and so on) or abnormal responses (increased body temperature, marked increase in perceived exertion), cut back and evaluate in greater detail. Fortunately, both of these outcomes are unusual. Usually there is clear improvement, and the responses are well within normal limits.

Several things that should be routinely checked appear on or can be calculated from the information provided by keeping an exercise log (see chapter 8, for example), such as speed, rating of perceived exertion, weekly exercise volume, average pulse, and so forth. Others are noted in the sample progress log (table 9.1) and should receive either a numerical value (weight, skinfolds, and glucose) or a "+," "0," or "–" rating (well-being, strength, and flexibility). Measuring skinfold

Table 9.1

Progress Log

Time/date	Weight	Well-being	Strength	Flexibility	Skinfolds	Glucose

thickness and blood glucose levels is not for everyone because it requires special expertise and equipment. When available, however, it usually provides helpful information.

During these two phases the dos and don'ts for this group are similar to those for the other two groups.

Dos and Don'ts

✓   Pay attention to environmental conditions.

✓   Pay attention to eating habits (to avoid low blood sugar).

✓   Stay well hydrated.

✓   Rest one hour for each hour of exercise (rest-activity cycling).

✓   Confirm pregnancy early.

✓   Seek medical help if abnormal symptoms develop.

✓   Don't get overheated.

✓   Don't get overtired.

✓   Don't travel to hotter climates or from sea level to high altitude.

Competitive Athletes

The attitudes and goals of the women in this group are very different from those of the other two. As a group, they are competitive, independent, headstrong, and feel deep down they know what's best for them and only want their health fitness and health care providers to confirm it. In addition, their performance goals and expectations usually exceed what will be possible at the time of conception and during pregnancy. For these reasons, I recommend that all women in this category develop a detailed and comprehensive program before attempting conception. They definitely should not do this alone; it is helpful if their coaches (or other health fitness instructor) and their health care providers are involved.

These professionals must gain the competitive athlete's trust and respect for the process to work. This is best done by using a no-nonsense approach that stresses logic, education, planning, and monitoring. If the appropriate relationship does not develop, then nothing productive will be accomplished, and the athlete and the initial providers should part company with the understanding that the athlete should try again with different personnel. If the relationship succeeds, then the athlete and her providers should make sure that the detail and depth of the program and monitoring matches the level of exercise performance and the difficulty of the set goals.

Education

The same material should be covered with this group as with the beginning and recreational athletes but the approach and attitude must be different. The goal for the recreational athlete was clarification and for the beginners to alleviate concern to ensure compliance. The major goal for the competitive athlete is to create enough genuine concern to ensure that the planned regimen is followed and not exceeded.

Clinician's Guide for Educating Competitive Exercisers About Pregnancy

Ensuring a competitive exerciser's compliance to a safe and effective exercise regimen requires an extremely detailed discussion of the reproductive issues involved when she maintains a serious training regimen throughout the various phases of the reproductive process. Approach the reproductive process from the same perspective that the athlete approaches training. This means a hard-nosed, no-nonsense, realistic approach. For example, set forth the goals the athlete wants to achieve, identify potential road blocks and the best way to avoid them, and figure out what steps are needed to meet these goals. Emphasize that success in reproduction will require the same commitment, flexibility, and occasional compromise as success in training and competition. When problems or conflicts arise, they must be resolved using the same logical approach as in the training arena.

Once you have covered the basics of the menstrual cycle, spend additional time detailing how stress in general and the physical and nutritional stresses of serious exercise training in particular can suppress ovulation if carried too far. The competitive athlete must hear, understand, and act upon the message that regular or at least semiregular ovulation is essential for conception.

A similar detailed discussion should address the potential adverse reproductive effects that could occur if a woman does not maintain the proper balance between the needs of the exercise program, the

cont'd ☞

reproductive process, and the rest of life while trying to conceive and during the early part of pregnancy. The four specific examples I like to use include the potential reproductive effects of overtraining, hyperthermia, dehydration, and serious competition. In short, the competitive athlete must also hear, understand, and act upon the message that balance, consistency, and attention to many little details is as, if not more, important for success in reproduction than in competition.

Stress the importance of monitoring multiple facets of both the exercise response and the reproductive process to determine where the appropriate balance point between exercise and reproductive function lies. Likewise, present material to ensure that each woman understands the rationale behind several additional important points. These points are as follows:

- This is not the time for a rapid increase in exercise volume.
- This is not the time for an all-out, sustained effort.
- This is not the time for high-altitude training.
- This is not the time for middle- or long-distance competitive events.

Set aside time to be sure that everyone understands all the important messages and that you have answered all their questions. The pace should be unhurried, and usually two sessions are required. In any case, a period of at least a few days should elapse between this initial educational component and the beginning of planning the details of the exercise and monitoring regimens to give each woman time to think through the information. This allows each to decide what she is or is not willing to do, which facilitates and helps focus the planning process.

Interactive Component

With this group, it's important to stress that if they are going to obtain the combined goals of maintaining a rigorous training schedule and getting pregnant simultaneously, then other aspects of their lifestyle must change; it's as simple as that. Now there are two priorities, not one, and success in both means something else is going to have to give. Specifically, competitive athletes trying to conceive and experiencing early pregnancy must pay more attention to maintaining adequate diet and hydration, getting enough nonphysical leisure activity to achieve a balance between rest and activity, and committing the time needed for monitoring and assessments.

Help the competitive athlete develop alternate strategies for achieving performance goals in case the symptoms and physical changes of pregnancy make it difficult to continue one or more aspects of the current training regimen. The success of the overall exercise program must be frequently assessed to determine if it's producing the desired effects on exercise performance, getting pregnant, and life in general. If it's not working in all areas, then either the goals or the plan needs to change—and change fast. That's the job of the coach and health care provider—to help the athlete deal quickly, realistically, and effectively with these challenges. In turn, the athlete should recognize that she must trust their judgment on these issues because usually she hasn't been pregnant before and doesn't know what's around the corner like they do.

Setting Goals

It's extremely important that the athlete and her health fitness and health care providers talk frankly and agree about what are and are not acceptable performance goals during these two phases of the reproductive process. Training goals are usually not the problem. All should readily agree on two main training goals: to maintain or improve basic fitness characteristics at both the whole body and cellular level and to improve sport-specific skills. The same is true for the reproductive goal of starting a healthy pregnancy.

The problem areas are all-out effort and serious competition. Unfortunately, there are no clear answers in these two areas. Anecdotal evidence suggests that at least some types of serious competition and all-out effort may be OK in well trained individuals (Clapp 1989a, 1994a; Cohen et al. 1989; Erdelyi 1962; Lotgering et al. 1991; Villarosa 1985). However, critical documentation of the physiological effects of these activities and long-term outcome data are lacking.

My personal approach to this is to begin by pointing out that it's not the competition that bothers me, it's the physiological effects that peaking, competition, and their attendant all-out, sustained efforts produce. Until we know more about it, it seems that it may be too risky; therefore, I discourage it.

I try, however, to be fair. If the athlete can be sure that she will avoid the four potential physiological threats to these phases of the reproductive process (anovulation, dehydration, hyperthermia, and hypoglycemia), then she probably will avoid others that are unknown as well. Under these circumstances, competition probably will be OK on a limited basis. So, my bottom line as the advisor and planner is this: Show me that you can achieve this level of performance in training without causing these problems, then I'll be willing to talk about competition seriously. Finally, I point out that the only way to determine if the athlete can or cannot train and compete without causing these problems is to take frequent measurements during the various training sessions.

I find this approach works most of the time. If it doesn't, the best approach is to be direct and suggest that the athlete pick another advisory team. To work together effectively as a team, the athlete must understand that the health care provider and health fitness instructor need to be as comfortable with the plan as she is.

Type of Exercise

I incorporate three components into the competitive athlete's training program: endurance, strength, and sport-specific skill training.

Endurance

Two types of endurance regimens (both overdistance and interval) are essential to maintaining and improving cardiovascular function, pulmonary function, tissue exchange, and fuel storage capacity for both the exercise and the reproductive process. I tend to rely on running because it's simple, low risk, and requires little equipment. During these phases, however, there's absolutely no reason to exclude things like in-line skating, cross-country skiing, stair machines, and so on. I find that swimmers do well swimming but that triathletes prefer to do something else. I reserve cycling for cyclists and triathletes because all the data discussed in earlier chapters suggest that weight-bearing exercise is most beneficial for obtaining the additive effects of pregnancy and exercise.

How much endurance training is enough? There's no right answer because the need is sport-specific. Everyone needs a base, but the needs of a sprinter or gymnast are much different from those of a mid- or long-distance runner. In well conditioned, regularly ovulating athletes, the best approach is probably to keep this component constant throughout these two phases. The volume should be similar to what it was before the woman began attempting pregnancy. My rationale for this approach is if you continue to do what the body is used to, you won't interfere with the critical reproductive factors. If you increase it very much, you might.

If there is evidence that the athlete is not ovulating regularly, a decision must be made about training volume: Should she cut back or not? That's not an easy question to answer correctly or quickly. Evaluating this issue correctly requires a relatively slow methodical approach of assessing the individual's overall situation. First, work together to identify all the various life stressors other than the training itself. Then, develop and follow a plan to determine if the reproductive problem can be resolved by changing the other life stressors rather than the exercise regimen. The following changes are usually helpful:

- Stabilize the lifestyle.
- Improve nutrition.
- Increase the time spent in nonphysical leisure time activity.
- Eliminate or reduce other stress-producing commitments and activities (committee work, overtime on the job, fund-raising, and the like).

If changes like these cannot be introduced or if they don't work in a reasonable time (two or three months), then the endurance component of the exercise program needs to be downsized. Cutting overdistance and interval training back by 25 percent is reasonable, and, if the endurance training is the culprit, a rapid reversal should occur. If there is no effect in three months, then it's probably not the exercise, and it's time for a detailed medical evaluation.

Strength

Weight training is essential to maintain or improve an athlete's strength during pregnancy. The specific program is usually highly individualized and sport-specific, and, as far as I've been able to ascertain, there is no reason to alter this component during the first two phases of the reproductive process. In the rare case in which an athlete doesn't have a strength-training program, develop one using machines. Initially, emphasize the upper body and extremities. Design the program to increase strength (many repetitions and sets) rather than muscle mass (maximal weight and limited repetitions).

Sport-Specific Skills

During these two phases there is no reason that skills training cannot continue at or above usual levels *unless* it creates problems with oxygenation, nutrition, hydration, or body temperature. For example, scuba diving to depths requiring decompression may disrupt embryonic oxygenation by causing "the bends" in specific growing tissues. Likewise, discourage "making weight" for ballet or gymnastics and insist on lots of fluids and occasional temperature checks during prolonged overdistance running.

Instruction and Safety

Once the exercise program is in place, it's time for the first of many equipment checks. With a high-volume training schedule, worn equipment is a constant hazard, and, depending on the activity, equipment checks should be conducted every two weeks to two months. The competitive athlete always profits from having her workouts observed on an intermittent basis. At these times, direct your attention toward improving biomechanics, surveying the training environment to be sure it's safe, and providing additional instruction.

<hr/>

Preventing dehydration, hyperthermia, and physical injury are key.

<hr/>

The other safety issues for this group include those issues discussed for beginners.

Monitoring

Intense monitoring is imperative for this group of athletes. During these early phases, it should focus on two things—the athlete's physiological responses to the exercise and ensuring that her reproductive function is normal. This will ensure both safety and progress. The evaluation of exercise performance should follow the same routine as it did before pregnancy.

<hr/>

Carefully monitor both the reproductive process and the physiological responses to training.

<hr/>

If a woman wants to get pregnant, she needs to ovulate regularly, so her ovulation pattern is an important reproductive function for her to monitor. There are several easy ways for her to tell if she ovulates regularly or not. First, does she have regular (26- to 30-day), normal (some premenstrual tension, some menstrual cramping, two or more days of flow) menstrual cycles? If so, she is regularly ovulating. Menstrual regularity coupled with premenstrual symptoms and cramping provide fairly conclusive evidence that ovulation occurred that cycle. Short-lived, midcycle, lower abdominal pain (often occurs when the egg is released) is another good sign that she is ovulating regularly. However, the two best indications are a midcycle rise in body temperature that persists until menses begins and a copious, clear, midcycle vaginal discharge that usually lasts 12 hours or so. The athlete can check the first by taking her temperature (preferably rectally) before arising each morning with a special ovulation thermometer. She should see an overnight rise in her temperature of 0.4 to 0.6 degrees, which persists for at least the next 12 days. If she pays careful attention, the second should be noticeable when she goes to the bathroom. I also recommend that she record her sexual activity on the chart she uses for her periods and her temperature to be sure she is having intercourse frequently around the time she is ovulating. If these things are OK and she doesn't get pregnant in three cycles, it's time to see the doctor.

Midcycle discharge and premenstrual cramps, coupled with a midcycle rise in temperature, indicate ovulation has occurred.

Once a woman suspects she's pregnant, it's wise to be sure that the pregnancy *dating* is accurate and to establish that it is progressing normally. There are two reasons this is important in this group. First, getting rid of uncertainty alleviates any anxiety the athlete may have about her reproductive capacity. Second, if problems arise in late pregnancy, one of the most important things in making decisions is knowing exactly how far along the pregnancy is. If you wait until then to figure it out it's easy to be off by three weeks or more. If you do it early, you'll be within a week. This takes an accurate last menstrual period (from her chart), a record of sexual activity during the cycle (from her chart as well), an early urine pregnancy test (first morning urine four days after the missed period), and an early abdominal ultrasound to confirm viability and measure the length of the baby (at five and one-half to six weeks postconception or seven and one-half to eight weeks post menses).

During these two periods, the thermal response to exercise is the most important exercise response to monitor. It's easy to do. The woman can take her temperature rectally or vaginally before and immediately after her hardest and longest workouts each week *before* she cools down. Under certain circumstances (workouts at the health club and Y are typically a problem), the athlete must plan the final stages of her workout carefully to assure that she can obtain the privacy she needs when she needs it. If she can afford it, she can buy a tympanic membrane thermometer, which allows her to obtain an accurate core temperature by inserting a sensor into her external ear canal. It's fast and easy, but expensive. (She shouldn't take her temperature orally; an oral temperature isn't accurate under these circumstances.) To be on the safe side, we usually measure the athletes' rectal temperature continuously with a flexible rectal thermistor (see figure 9.2). This is especially true for competitive swimmers because the temperature of the pool makes a real difference. If it's too warm (greater than 82 degrees Fahrenheit) and they are doing over a 4,000-yard workout, they may get too hot. Similar portable devices are available but they really are not practical outside of a research setting.

The upper limit of what's OK for the thermal response isn't known. Based on our experience, however, it seems that a rise of up to 1.6 degrees centigrade (about 3 degrees Fahrenheit) or a peak temperature up to 102 degrees Fahrenheit is not associated with abnormal outcome. However, if the athlete either exceeds or is consistently at these levels, the wisest course is to abruptly alter the thermal characteristics of the training environment (time of day, air conditioning, and so on) or the duration of the extremely intense portion of the workouts (usually the intervals). If that doesn't work right away, a few other environmental modifications can be tried (intermittent drenching with cool water from a hose, fans, and the like). If those measures don't work, then the sensible and safe thing to do is alter the training regimen a bit more. The easiest additional change is to split up the parts of the workout that precipitate the problem.

The final three responses that need to be monitored are fluid loss, blood glucose, and sense of well-being. Monitoring fluid loss keeps track of the extent to which the athlete depletes her blood volume, which reflects the level of circulatory stress imposed (the fall in blood flow to the womb). It's easy to measure; all she needs to do is strip down, wipe off, and weigh herself before and after her hardest workouts (sweat-laden clothes weigh a lot). At this time, it's probably wise to keep weight loss below three pounds per workout. Remember, in early pregnancy, the woman is low on circulating blood volume anyway, and a water bottle should be her constant companion.

The blood glucose level reflects the availability of energy for both the growth process and the exercise. Starting early in pregnancy, the liver wants to direct all the sugar to fat, so it's difficult to get it to release the sugar for other things. Therefore, unless the exercise is quite strenuous (which increases stress hormones that stimulate glucose release), blood sugar can fall rapidly, especially during and after low-intensity, overdistance training. The response gets worse as pregnancy

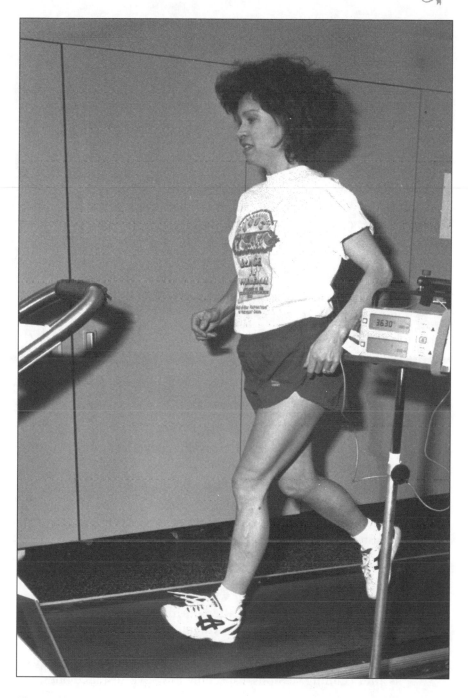

Figure 9.2   Monitoring the thermal approach to exercise in early pregnancy.

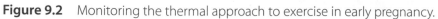

advances, so it's a good idea to start monitoring it as soon as conception occurs. The athlete can do it herself by pricking her finger with a metal stylet, squeezing a drop of her blood onto a glucose strip, and reading it with a portable monitor like diabetics use. After awhile, she'll have a good idea when to check it by the way she feels. A reasonable goal is to maintain the level above 55 to 60 milligrams per deciliter.

A sense of well-being is the best check for evidence of overtraining in early pregnancy. The athlete should ask herself twice a week how she feels in the morning, then answer from a mental and physical perspective. If the answer is "great" or "pretty good," she's home free. If it's "I'm sore" or "not so good," then it's time to reevaluate.

Competitive athletes who are trying to get pregnant or who are in the early stages of a pregnancy should follow these rules when exercising.

Dos and Don'ts

✓ *Pay attention to environmental conditions; specifically, avoid hot, humid environments and poor ventilation.* The competitive athlete should check her thermal response periodically and any time she feels hotter than she thinks she should. To date, we've only been able to identify one truly high-risk situation. That occurs when competitive athletes do extremely intense interval sets in the usual health club or gym environment. If they perform exercises that use extensive muscle mass (plyometrics and versa climbing are two examples), core temperature climbs rapidly and can exceed 102 degrees if they continue the activity for more than 15 or 20 minutes.

✓ *Stay well hydrated and salt replete by drinking water regularly all day long as well as while exercising.* Clear urine is a sure sign of adequate hydration. Not exercising strenuously unless the urine is clear is a good rule to follow.

✓ *Eat frequently and well.* Adjust caloric intake based on morning weight. This is definitely not the time to lose weight; if anything, put on a little weight while attempting pregnancy and at least a pound a week thereafter during pregnancy. Eating two or three hours before training will minimize the exercise-induced fall in blood sugar. Likewise, at this training level, the athlete should begin supplemental carbohydrate intake during as well as after training sessions, especially long overdistance ones.

✓ *Stay away from fad diets and supervitamins.* Regular supplements are OK, but high doses of several (vitamin A is the big offender) are strongly associated with congenital malformations.

✓ *Follow the rest-activity cycle plan.* For competitive athletes, adequate rest is extremely important; however, it's easy to let other things interfere. Several tricks may help. If a woman can get used to taking an afternoon nap, it really helps, and the symptoms of fatigue in early pregnancy make it easier to establish that as a daily pattern. A nap coupled with an early to bed, early to rise policy ensures the athlete is on an ideal schedule for the pregnancy and the training. Another approach is to use leisure time to explore other areas of interest. The library is an excellent source of good books and videotapes on almost any topic, and most athletes are interested in several areas other than exercise (at this point all kinds of issues relating to childcare are new and interesting as well). Table and word games, movies, and TV are additional options as are many social group activities. Good sources for group activities include other athletes and one or more of the local athletic clubs.

✓ *Remember, the best time to conceive (and thus the best timing for sexual activity) is around midcycle.* Competitive athletes have likely heard all the rumors about athletes and infertility, too, and many do miss periods now and then. The sooner they get pregnant, the more relaxed they'll be and that will make everything a lot easier.

✓ *Confirm the pregnancy and see the doctor or midwife early.*

✓ *Use common sense.*

✓ *Don't train at altitudes higher than 7,500 feet.* Exercise aside, there are clear suggestions that pregnancies in women accustomed to sea level do not do well if the women go up to high altitude and stay there in early, mid-, or late pregnancy (Falk 1983).

✓ *Don't ignore symptoms that may indicate a significant problem.* They include localized, persistent pain, vaginal bleeding, and a sudden change in feelings of well-being.

✓ *Don't lead an erratic lifestyle.* Focus on the two important issues of the moment and build the rest of life around them.

Needs of Other Exercising Women

As mentioned earlier, exercise prescription for women with underlying disease is beyond the scope of this book. The design and conduct of the exercise program should be approached as a team effort (the woman, her multiple health care providers, and a fitness trainer) and preferably as part of a study protocol or program because not a lot is known in this area. Studies are now starting to examine the potential preventive and/or therapeutic value of exercise in a variety of disease states in pregnancy (hypertension, gestational diabetes, and premature birth are the best examples). But it's going to be a while before there is much information available. Right now we know a little about some of the detrimental effects of exercise with many types of underlying disease, and most of that has been learned by trial and error. At any rate, until we know a lot more, most women in this group will need highly individualized and detailed attention.

Summary

Basically, the first two phases of the reproductive cycle are a time for developing an understanding of what is going on and why it's important to do certain exercises and follow certain guidelines and not others. Specifically, they're a time for evaluation and preparation for what's to come in all three groups. Although the specific needs of various women are different, there are common threads in the approaches and the emphasis placed on the different components of the appropriate exercise programs.

   The common problem areas that arise when regular exercise and reproduction are combined include maintaining reproductive rhythms, relieving anxiety, and avoiding stress, fatigue, and excessive physiological responses to the exercise. The common solutions are paying attention to detail and using a common sense approach to balance the needs of both within the context of the individual's lifestyle. The important reproductive details involve regular ovulation, fertilization, and normal early development. The important exercise details include maintaining or improving performance without developing hyperthermia, dehydration, or hypoglycemia (low blood sugar). Additional important factors include nutrition, adequate rest, and maintaining a personal sense of well-being. These will continue to be important. The next chapter deals with what to expect, do, and not do during mid- and late pregnancy.

CHAPTER 10

Mid- and Late Pregnancy

id- and late pregnancy are times of continual change for the mother and baby. Nothing stays the same, and when you add exercise to the mix it can get tricky. So it's logical that the planning and design of an exercise program focus on serially evaluating responses to both the exercise and the pregnancy in order to balance their needs as the pregnancy evolves.

I begin the chapter by noting the important physiological things going on during mid- and late pregnancy. I discuss the contraindications to continuing regular exercise during mid- and late pregnancy. Then I discuss the details of the exercise program itself because the rest of the chapter deals with balance, adaptation, and compromise, and I don't want anyone to forget that there are circumstances when it is in the best interest of the mother, the baby, or both to stop exercising. I spend the remainder of the chapter on what is important for both the exercise and the pregnancy, what to do, what not to do, and why.

Physiological Function in Midpregnancy

For the baby this is what I call the *meat and potatoes phase*. He or she grows and develops rapidly into a miniature person, but functional maturation doesn't occur until later in the pregnancy. This means that the baby is dependent on its placenta and mother for functional integrity as well as a good supply of oxygen and nutrients. In addition, there are two twists that make it more interesting. The placenta regulates the balance between the needs of the mother for exercise and the needs of the baby for growth (Clapp 1994b), yet regular exercise over this time period also improves the growth and functional capacity of the placenta (see chapters 2 and 3) (Clapp and Rizk 1992; Jackson et al. 1995). So, the stress of exercise stimulates the development of the organ that ultimately protects and balances the needs of the mother and baby.

Thus, indexes of the placenta's functional capability can be used to determine if the pregnancy is in appropriate balance with the exercise program and proceeding normally. For research purposes, this can be measured precisely (Clapp 1994b), but the techniques are complicated and require special equipment. There is, however, one practical way that works well. Simply monitor the placenta's functional product—the growth rate of the baby. If the placenta is working very well, the baby will grow rapidly. If it's average functionally, the baby will grow at an average rate, and, if there is a problem, the baby will grow either slowly or not at all. Fortunately, the baby's growth rate is sensitive, so a small change in function causes a noticeable change in growth. As a result, it's an excellent way to check that the balance is right and the pregnancy is proceeding normally.

For the mother this is the "I've never felt better" phase of the reproductive process. If that is not the case a thorough evaluation is indicated. The symptoms of early pregnancy are over and the adaptations are almost complete. She usually feels well and has an unbelievable amount of get up and go. In practical terms, this means the major problem will be making sure that she does not exceed her recommended training regimen.

Physiological Function in Late Pregnancy

For the baby, this is the time when all its organs functionally mature so it can deal with life outside the uterus effectively. He or she starts to develop behavioral patterns, cycles from one behavioral state to another, and is awake on a regular basis. Indeed, many feel that this is when the baby responds to what is going on outside the uterus (especially sound and vibration). They believe if the parents control what goes on outside, they can enhance neurological development and influence personality. In practical terms, the development of behavioral patterns means that the baby's responses to a variety of things (including exercise) can be used to evaluate his or her condition.

In late pregnancy, the woman's focus shifts from training to preparing for the birth.

For the mother, this is a time she wants to be over. All of a sudden, she's much larger than she wants to be, is tired of being kicked by the baby, doesn't sleep well, and wonders if the baby is OK and what labor and delivery will be like. As a result, her attention turns away from herself to prepare for the labor, the birth, and the new baby. Thus, as the time for delivery approaches, the exercise program may become a secondary priority. Most women by this point in the pregnancy, however, know that exercise makes them feel better and that they stand a better chance of an early, uncomplicated birth if they continue exercising. This means that most women's motivation to exercise remains high until delivery and therefore sticking to a safe and effective exercise regimen is not a problem. So, if exercising women are a ball of energy in midpregnancy and remain motivated up to term, it makes sense to shift gears now and pay attention to the reasons why they should stop.

Contraindications to Exercise

Of course the basic contraindications to exercise during mid- and late pregnancy are the same as those discussed in chapter 8—injury, illness, heavy vaginal bleeding, and pain. However, there are a few additional ones to watch for at this time. I divide them into two categories: absolute and relative contraindications.

Absolute Contraindications

The first absolute contraindication is recurrent, light vaginal bleeding that originates inside the womb. The last point is important because local changes in the tissues at the mouth of the womb can be the culprit. So, it's important that the woman be examined by her physician or midwife during a bleeding episode to pinpoint the source.

If the bleeding is coming from the mouth of the womb or vaginal wall, it's usually OK to continue exercise. If it's coming from inside the womb, however, it usually means that the placenta is in the wrong place (near or over the mouth of the womb), separating at its edges from the wall of the womb, or undergoing progressive vascular damage. None of these are good signs, all require intensive medical evaluation, and all are aggravated by physical activity. If such a problem progresses, it can lead to premature labor, catastrophic hemorrhage, and sometimes even death. There's really no choice. The woman must stop exercising, even if it's only a little bit of bleeding!

The second absolute contraindication is rupture of the membranes that surround the baby before the onset of labor. It doesn't make any difference whether this happens at term or earlier in the pregnancy. Under these circumstances, the motions of both weight-bearing and most types of nonweight-bearing exercise can cause the umbilical cord to slip beside the baby's head and shoulders where it can get compressed. Remember that the placenta is the baby's lung, so compressing the umbilical cord is like choking the baby, and, of course, that's not good. In addition, when the membranes rupture well before term, the motion associated with weight-bearing exercise can stimulate labor when it should be stopped as well as increase the chance of infection due to bacteria ascending from the vagina into the womb.

The third absolute contraindication is evidence that the woman has either started or may soon start labor well ahead of schedule (before the last month of pregnancy). When these symptoms appear, the baby is at risk, so it's wise to stop exercising. There's no problem deciding that this is the right thing to do if the woman suddenly starts labor, goes to the hospital, and drugs are used successfully to stop it. But often it's not that easy. After the start of the seventh month, it's usual and quite normal to have contractions that increase in frequency every week. Occasionally, they get strong and regular enough to make the woman (and sometimes the doctor) think she's in labor when she's not (false labor). Exercise complicates the matter because it stimulates uterine activity, and women notice a progressive increase in cramps during exercise in late pregnancy. This is normal, and usually there's no problem, but how does a woman tell for sure?

In our experience, it appears that this crampy response to exercise is a valuable screening tool for identifying women at risk for preterm labor. As long as the cramps stop shortly after the woman stops exercise, there's no problem. However, if they persist for more than 20 to 30 minutes after the woman stops exercise, true labor may not be far off. In the individual case, the only way to be sure is for the doctor or midwife to do periodic internal examinations to determine if there is evidence that the mouth of the womb is slowly thinning out and dilating ahead of schedule. If that occurs, no matter how well the woman feels, she should stop exercising. If it doesn't happen, there's no cause for concern.

The fourth is evidence that the uterus or womb is not structurally normal. When this occurs, there is a much greater chance that the woman will go into labor ahead of schedule. Sometimes, there is evidence at the first medical examination that the mouth of the womb has been damaged or hasn't developed properly (common in women whose mothers took D.E.S when they were pregnant; see chapter 1). Usually, however, there is no advance warning, and the abnormality is not diagnosed until a detailed medical evaluation is done after an initial premature birth. If there is any evidence of structural abnormalities of the uterus, it is prudent to stop exercise early in any subsequent pregnancy because the evidence suggests that, in this specific situation, rest may prevent premature labor from happening again.

The fifth absolute contraindication is an acute illness or a problem with the pregnancy that the doctor feels should be treated by restricting activity. Although these cases are not always clear-cut, a pregnant woman should follow her doctor's guidelines. Two main problems with pregnancy that fall into this category are concern that the baby is growing too slowly and evidence of elevated blood pressure with excessive fluid retention. Traditionally, both are treated with rest.

Relative Contraindications

For healthy women, many of the other contraindications to exercise are relative, not absolute. The two most controversial are twin pregnancy (multiple-birth pregnancies beyond twins are discussed below) and a history of a going into labor before the last month (see the synopsis of current guidelines in chapter 8). The reasons some professionals recommend that women who carry twins decrease their activity are that labor with twins often starts before term and the demands for growth are much greater with two than they are with one. When researchers look at this issue with a critical eye, however, they note that preterm labor happens with twins whether you cut back on activity or not. Therefore, I think the logical thing to do is for a woman pregnant with twins to be followed closely by her health care provider while exercising in late pregnancy. If evidence develops that preterm birth may occur, she should stop exercising; if it doesn't, she can continue. The same thing is true for concern about the growth rates of the twins in utero. If growth rates are normal, continuing to exercise is fine; if growth rates fall off, stop.

To date, we've had six women in our studies that conceived twins. Five decided to continue exercise, and the outcomes were all OK. One of the five was advised to stop in midpregnancy because of some early changes in the mouth of the womb. She did and delivered healthy twins at term. In another of the five, the pregnancy went well until the eighth month when one of the babies stopped growing; the woman's doctor decided to deliver her ahead of schedule. Both babies were in good condition at birth and have done well. In the other three cases, the pregnancies were entirely normal, and the women continued to exercise and delivered healthy, normally grown twins at term. The woman who stopped regular exercise as soon as a twin pregnancy was diagnosed delivered uneventfully three weeks before her due date.

What about triplet pregnancy or those rare ones with four or more? Unfortunately, these pregnancies usually are complicated by multiple maternal and fetal problems and extremely premature births are common. Because of these multiple problems the health care focus is directed at maintaining adequate growth of all the babies and doing everything possible to prolong the pregnancy. As a result, current practice is to restrict maternal activity even though its true value in enhancing growth and prolonging the pregnancy is not known. Until more is known, my advice is to follow the recommendations of the health care team.

Women who have delivered early in a previous pregnancy also may continue exercising into mid- and late pregnancy under the supervision of their health care provider, unless there is evidence of structural damage to the womb. Most of the other relative contraindications involve underlying maternal diseases (heart, lungs, endocrine glands, bone, or muscle). As mentioned earlier, I recommend an individualized, team approach among health care providers, fitness instructors, and the pregnant woman. Now, we'll continue with what to do and not do for the majority of women who can safely continue to exercise throughout mid- and late pregnancy.

Prescribing Exercise

The specifics of developing an exercise program for women in mid- and late pregnancy are no different for the beginner than they are for the competitive athlete. They differ only in the amount of surveillance required to balance the intensity of the training program with the needs of the pregnancy. As I've covered the general and specific recommendations for beginning, recreational, and competitive athletes in chapters

8 and 9, I'll approach mid- and late pregnancy with one guideline at a time, discussing what is necessary for each group.

Education

At this point in the pregnancy, the educational effort for beginning, recreational, and competitive athletes should focus on four areas. First, they all need to know what lies ahead. Therefore, they will benefit from a discussion, pictorial book, or video dealing with the sequential growth and development of the baby and the changes that the remainder of pregnancy will produce in both mind and body. This information provides the necessary background for the last two areas—the effect the rest of pregnancy will have on exercise performance and the effects that continuing exercise will have on them, their babies, and the course and outcome of their pregnancies. The information should be the same for all three groups (see part II, chapters 3-7).

Focus the educational component on growth and development of the baby, maternal changes, and the interactions between the pregnancy and the exercise.

Monitoring

Throughout this phase of the reproductive process, continue to monitor the acute and chronic responses to exercise. They both involve the same measures we've discussed earlier, but now they can be expanded to assess the baby's response as well. It's the findings in this area that confirm that the balance between the exercise and the reproductive process is where it should be. It's simple. All that needs to be done is to periodically check the well-being of both mother and baby. If both are doing well, the balance is right. If there's evidence of a change in either, the balance needs to be fine-tuned.

Assess Acute Responses

The acute responses of the mother and baby to a typical training session should be periodically assessed to be sure that the exercise is not creating an acute problem that might have some chronic effects (poor

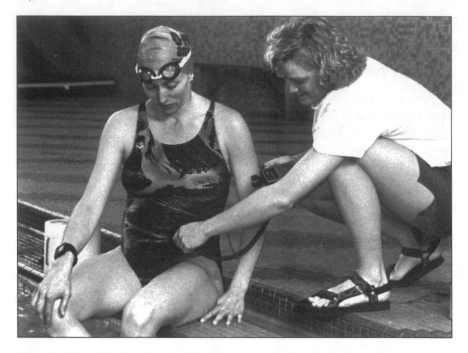

Figure 10.1 Monitoring the fetal heart rate response to swimming.

growth, brain damage, or the like). The frequency and extent of the evaluation will differ among the three groups, but the approach should be the same. Focus on the changes in maternal temperature, hydration, blood glucose concentration, and performance level, but add an evaluation of the baby's heart rate and behavioral responses as well. As shown in figure 10.1, it's quick and easy to do.

> In mid-and late pregnancy, focus on the thermal, metabolic, and fetal heart rate responses.

The beginners require evaluation every four to six weeks. The extent of evaluation should depend on the changes in their exercise performance—the more exercise, the more in-depth the evaluation. Thus, the evaluation can range from checking the baby's heartbeat and activity before and after and asking a few questions (Do you feel hot when you start sweating? Do you feel hungry or weak? and so on) to that required for the most serious athletes.

The competitive athlete should be evaluated every two weeks and her most demanding workouts (both duration and intensity) should be monitored. Special equipment is usually necessary, so the evaluation should be done routinely in an exercise testing laboratory or sports center. Ideally, her core temperature should be monitored continuously before, during, and for 10 minutes after exercise using a flexible rectal thermistor (see figure 9.2; Clapp 1991). If that's not possible, then the athlete should check her temperature after the most intense portion of the workout as well as before and after the entire session. She can do this rectally using an electronic thermometer, or, if the equipment is available, a measure of tympanic membrane temperature using one of the newer ear thermometers is more convenient and perfectly acceptable. If her temperature exceeds the limits set (see chapter 9), she should change the pattern, environment, or the intensity of these workouts.

Measure weight before and after the session as well as fluid loss from the vascular compartment (hematocrit or plasma protein concentration) to assess fluid shifts. Measure blood glucose concentration before and after exercise as well. The upper limits for weight loss, rise in hematocrit, and fall in blood glucose should be set between three and four pounds, 15 percent or four to six points, and 25 milligrams percent, respectively. Check intensity and efficiency of performance by measuring workload, oxygen consumption, perceived level of exertion, and blood lactate levels. Changes in the last three without a change in the first suggest that the workload needs to increase if efficiency is improved or decrease if it is not.

In all competitive athletes, it is important to monitor the fetal heart rate and behavioral responses to exercise (figure 10.1). If the magnitude of the responses exceeds the limits set, use ultrasound to check movement, behavioral state, breathing motions, and placental size as well. A normal response in this group would be fetal heart rate increases of 10 to 25 beats per minute in midpregnancy and up to 35 beats per minute in late pregnancy. A decrease, no increase, or a greater increase on two consecutive occasions suggests that oxygen delivery may not be ideal, indicating a need for the more detailed ultrasound evaluation. If that can't be done, then an abrupt 10 to 20 percent decrease in exercise intensity and duration is indicated. If the problem recurs, a more detailed evaluation is mandatory.

The monitoring requirements for the recreational athlete who is increasing her performance level lies somewhere between the first two. Like the beginner, she should be evaluated every four to six weeks. In my opinion, the minimum evaluation should include the maternal blood glucose and thermal responses, assessment of progress with her level of physical performance, and the fetal heart rate response.

Assess Maternal Well-Being

The things to check in this category are all familiar and apply to all three groups. They include the following:

- A subjective assessment of feelings of fatigue, discomfort, and satisfaction with performance
- Weight gain and, possibly, fat accretion
- Hydration status
- Rest-activity cycling
- The relationship between performance level and perceived exertion

If a woman subjectively feels OK (see figures 10.2 and 10.3), rests appropriately, keeps her urine clear, and gains adequate weight, she can usually maintain or increase her current exercise program. If not, then she should make appropriate adjustments in either other lifestyle behaviors or the exercise regimen. In either case, a two- or three-point change in perceived exertion is a clear indication that the level of performance should change. If perceived exertion falls, the regimen should increase, and vice versa.

Assess Fetal Well-Being

Only the woman's health care provider can check some of the signs of fetal well-being. However, subjective sensations of uterine activity and the baby's activity patterns during the day are valuable, and the woman should pay special attention to the effects of the exercise sessions on them. A change in either is a valuable warning sign. When a baby gets in trouble, he or she decreases activity throughout the day to conserve energy. After exercise, the baby should move several times within the first 20 to 30 minutes and uterine contractility should quiet down quickly. Progressive changes in abdominal size indicate that the baby is growing, and the baby's heart rate response is a good index of oxygenation.

Focus pregnancy monitoring on growth, activity, uterine irritability, and the baby's heart rate response to exercise.

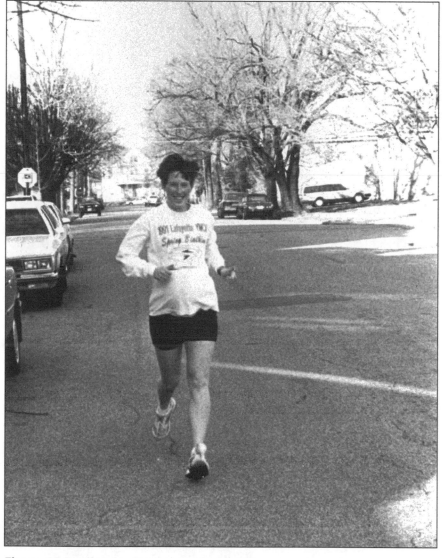

Figure 10.2   Training run in late pregnancy.

A health care provider usually monitors the adequacy of growth in detail by measuring the increase in the size of the uterus and feeling the baby every two to four weeks. If there's any question, the health care provider usually requests an ultrasound exam for detailed measurement of the size of the baby and placenta and the amount of amniotic fluid. He or she can also check the mouth of the womb periodically to be sure that the changes preceding labor are not occurring too early. If there is a serious question about fetal well-being, the health care provider may also request tests of fetal heart rate responses, breathing activity, and behavioral state cycling.

Usually, I check these things in beginners by asking them if their baby is moving as much this week as last, if the doctor was happy with the baby's growth at her last visit, and so on. I recommend, however, that both the competitive athlete and the health fitness instructor or trainer talk directly with the woman's health care provider (remember the don't ask, don't tell problem discussed in chapter 1?). All concerned should be sure that the midwife or doctor feels that everything, including the baby's growth rate, is entirely normal, and that he or she is aware of the competitive athlete's training regimen. In the recreational athlete, I recommend taking a middle-of-the-road approach. This approach centers on having the recreational athlete talk with her providers about everything that's happening in the pregnancy that might relate to her exercise. The following are examples of appropriate questions:

- Does the doctor think the baby is growing normally?
- How big will the baby be?
- How much uterine activity is normal?
- Should the baby be this active?

Modifying the Training Regimen

How much exercise is enough? The results of the monitoring provide the answer. As long as the acute responses to exercise stay within the prescribed limits and maternal and fetal well-being are OK, the woman can progressively increase or simply maintain her exercise regimen. As illustrated in figure 10.3, this is usually the case in fit women who continue a vigorous training regimen five or more times each week. If this is not the case, however, then it's time to modify or cut back. The approach is straightforward and similar in all three groups. The other consideration that comes up occasionally in the competitive athlete is safety.

Either a change in well-being or abnormal physiological responses indicate that the training regimen needs to be modified.

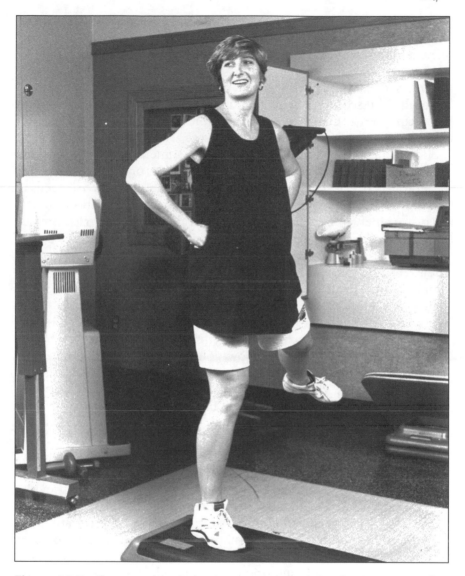

Figure 10.3 Step aerobics in late pregnancy: Stepping for 60 minutes, five times a week, is fine as long as everything is A-OK.

The most common situation is that the pregnancy is progressing normally and the acute responses are OK, but the woman's sense of well-being is not the best. This usually requires minimal modification (change in rest-activity patterns, training emphasis, exercise type, or the like). If the symptoms of overtraining occur, the usual culprit is either worn equipment or an incorrect balance between rest and activity. If they're OK, the workload should be decreased by 10 to 20 percent, another activity should be substituted, or the emphasis should be changed (move away from strength to endurance training, eliminate intervals, decrease sport-specific activities, or the like). If the problem is localized discomfort or pain and it's not an equipment or support problem, then a substitute activity is indicated (water running, weight machines, stair climbers, and ski machines are all helpful).

If both the mother and baby are OK but some aspect of the training elicits a response that either exceeds the set limits or is unusual in some other way (cardiac arrhythmia, for example), then the exercise needs to change. For example, we've noticed that competitive athletes who perform extremely intense forms of interval training (plyometrics, bounding, and vertical climbers are the three culprits we've identified so far) overwhelm their enhanced ability to dissipate heat and can quickly raise their rectal temperatures over 102 degrees. The solution to this problem is to shorten and break up the intervals. The other common problem is low blood sugar during and after a prolonged, low-intensity workout. The woman can usually handle this by changing the timing of the exercise relative to food intake (three hours without food before starting) coupled with frequent low-volume carbohydrate intake during and immediately after the training session. Fresh or dried fruit and a sports drink are excellent sources during the workout. Afterward, things like granola, a sandwich made from whole grain bread containing lots of veggies, a big bran muffin, or several pieces of fresh fruit are good choices.

Fortunately, the baby's status is rarely questionable when the mother feels well and all the acute maternal responses are OK. If there is a problem it usually is picked up by the woman's health care provider and, as discussed earlier, most often involves concern over the baby's rate of growth or the possibility of preterm delivery. Although the false positive rate for both is high, it's still important to follow the provider's advice. Look at it this way, if he or she is wrong, no harm is done, but if he or she is right and their opinion is ignored, it could be disastrous.

Comfort

Late in pregnancy appropriate support of the abdomen and breasts during exercise makes all the difference. For abdominal comfort, the key is upward lift and mild compression on the lower abdomen, which lifts the womb off the pelvic bones and stabilizes it. This relieves the pressure on the bladder and pelvic bones and minimizes sudden changes in the tension on the supporting ligaments. Snug overgirths help, and there are several commercial belts available for less than 20 dollars that do a good job. They are advertised in many magazines targeting active women, and you can purchase them at most stores specializing in maternity apparel. They're made out of elasticized fabric with Velcro attachments that let you individualize the position and tension of the belt (see figure 10.4). The other thing that works well is a wide Ace bandage wrapped snugly over the hips and down under the womb. However, especially in tall women, it can slip and require frequent readjustment. The key to stabilizing the breasts is compression against the chest wall, not lift. Wearing two athletic bras (on top of one another) helps. If that's not enough, try wrapping an Ace bandage around the chest, over the first but under the second bra.

Support and stabilize the breasts and abdomen.

Continue floor exercises, stretching, and weight training. Although the American College of Obstetricians and Gynecologists guidelines suggest limiting the range of motion and avoiding the supine position, I have not found objective information indicating that these really need to change during mid- or late pregnancy. The only exception is late in pregnancy when it is physically impossible for the woman to lie, let alone perform exercise, in the prone (stomach down) position. Floor exercises on the back appear to be OK unless the woman gets dizzy or the fetal heart rate response is abnormal. If one of these problems occurs, the woman should turn on her left side. Remember, lying still under the weight of the womb is what causes the problem, because the weight of the enlarged womb compresses and blocks the large vein that returns blood to the heart (inferior vena cava). My experience indicates that as long as the legs and torso are moving, interference with blood flow back to the heart should not be a problem. The weight training, floor exercises, and stretching keep a woman flexible and strong, which helps posture, reduces musculoskeletal stress, and makes her feel a lot better.

Safety Considerations

Both experience in other areas and deficiencies in our knowledge indicate that sometimes during pregnancy it's wise to be careful about

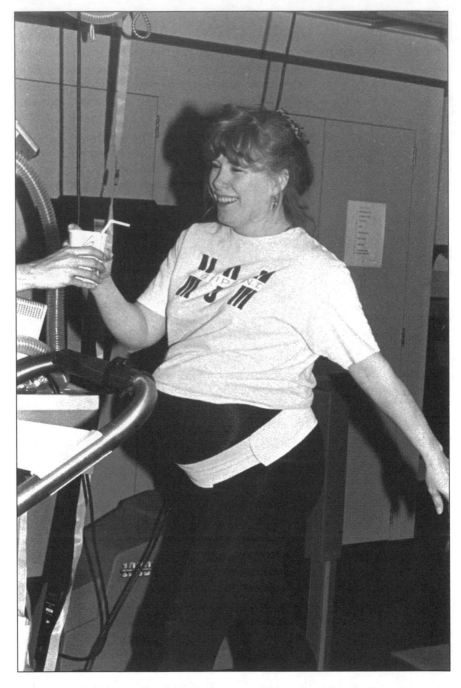

Figure 10.4   Abdominal support helps relieve pelvic pressure.

exercise. Most of these questions involve the risks of abdominal trauma, acute changes in the gas tensions in the air we breathe, and competitive sport. When confronted by the ardent enthusiast, my approach is that the limitations of pregnancy are quite minimal. If you can stay fit and have fun doing something else, why take the risk? I deal with the first two risks here and discuss competition in the next section.

Avoid high altitude, scuba diving, competition, and situations
with a high risk of abdominal trauma.

Information from automobile accidents and other types of trauma clearly demonstrate that once the womb becomes an abdominal organ (14 to 16 weeks after the last menstrual period), both penetrating and blunt abdominal trauma can damage the pregnancy. So it's common sense for a woman to modify or eliminate performing recreational exercise that carries a high risk of abdominal trauma (horseback riding, some aspects of gymnastics, high-speed water skiing, serious rock climbing, hockey, or the like).

Both high-altitude sport (climbing and skiing) and scuba diving alter the tensions of the gases in the air we breathe. At high altitude (9,000 feet and above), the level of oxygen decreases to the point at which acute exposure can cause significant illness (high-altitude sickness). It usually does cause symptoms of fatigue, shortness of breath, and minor sleep disturbances in most of us above that level. So, my attitude is why bother—we can perform both sports at lower altitudes anyway.

In scuba diving, the deeper the dive, the greater the increase in the tension of nitrogen as well as oxygen in the blood. That's why, pregnant or not, one must avoid diving too deep (nitrogen narcosis is common about 120 feet down). In particular, pregnant women should not dive deeper than 16 feet without doubling their decompression time (the bends occur if you don't). If the diver ascends to the surface too fast, bubbles of nitrogen form in tissues where the blood flow is low because at high pressures it can't get out of the tissues fast enough. It's painful and can cause permanent damage. During pregnancy, the question is "What about the diffusion out of the baby?" Not only does the nitrogen have to get out of the baby's tissues, it also must get back across the placenta. Right now we don't know if the decompression sequences should be altered to allow additional time for the compressed gases to get out of the baby and across the placenta. Thus, it seems prudent either to avoid diving at or near a depth that requires decompression or, at the very least, to extend decompression times by 50 percent.

Competition

We've discussed the issue of competing in sports late in pregnancy already. This is not typically an issue with the beginner. It occasionally comes up with the recreational athlete, but it's usually in the context of a fun run or a team event (relay, one leg of a team marathon or triathlon, or the like). My approach is, if the competition is for fun, it's OK, *if the woman takes it easy and it doesn't require her to exceed her usual training volume.* If her attitude toward the event is more serious she probably should not compete. This approach is safe because the serial monitoring done confirms that it's OK, as long as she doesn't exceed her usual level of performance.

The issue often comes up in mid- and even late pregnancy with the competitive athlete, and the approach should be exactly the same. If it's for fun, OK. If it's serious, no way! There's still a problem, however. It's hard for a competitive athlete to have fun when she's way back in the pack, holding back, and people are passing her. She feels fine, and all of a sudden she forgets, gets competitive, and breaks the rules. For this reason, I try to discourage competitive athletes from competing at this time. If that doesn't work, I meet with her, get out her records, and set reasonable performance limits (duration, speed, and intensity). Then I simply hope she follows them.

Summary

Before we go on to continuing an exercise program after the birth (chapter 11), let's go over some important points one more time. First, check equipment and the exercise environment. Many answers to symptoms and unanticipated responses are found here. I encourage using new equipment and ancillary protective gear. Surfaces should be even, and, during exercise, a pregnant woman should avoid hot and humid conditions. Maintaining hydration and an appropriate pattern of food intake are essential. The water bottle should be the pregnant woman's best friend, and, if she eats right, low blood sugar and weight gain should not be problems. Remember, weight gain and fat accumulation are the best index of adequate caloric intake until late in pregnancy. Fatigue is one of the pregnant woman's worst enemies. In mid- and late pregnancy, it's best avoided by decreasing unnecessary commitments and gradually including more rest in the day. Finally, remember the golden rule—when all else fails, use common sense.

CHAPTER 11

Postpartum

After the birth of a baby, life gets more complicated. Once there's a baby, there's a lot more going on day and night. Getting to know the baby is fun and rewarding, but it takes lots of time, and unless a woman is careful, she'll have no personal time. If it's not the baby, it's relatives, friends, or someone from work calling or visiting. Then there are the birth announcements, going back to work, and so forth. Where does exercise fit in—or does it? First, let's discuss the physiological changes that occur after the birth.

Physiological Changes of Exercise and Lactation During the Postpartum Period

In our experience, over 95 percent of the women we study successfully breast-feed their offspring, and we have noticed that some of the physiological changes of lactation influence exercise prescription in one way or another. These include effects on fluid and caloric balance, hormonal function, and breast size and mobility.

After the birth, nipple stimulation from infant suckling initiates and regulates milk production through several mechanisms. The more suckling, the more milk, and vice versa. As a result, milk production is largely regulated by the caloric needs of an infant as he or she grows and develops. These fluid and caloric demands increase steadily during infancy; they must be met by increases in maternal intake and soon exceed those of many exercise programs (10 to 15 ounces and 300 to 400 kilocalories at birth, increasing more than twofold by one year of age). Experience has shown that women who exercise regularly while they are breast-feeding spontaneously increase their caloric intakes to the appropriate level (Dewey et al. 1994; Little et al. 1994) but the same is not true for fluid intake. Therefore, women who wish to combine exercise with breast-feeding should be aware that to avoid volume depletion and poor performance in both areas, they must drink adequate quantities of fluid at regular intervals throughout the day. What is an adequate quantity for one woman may not be adequate for another, so I recommend that women use urine color as a guide: the clearer the urine, the better hydrated she is.

The stimulus of suckling also initiates hormonal changes in the mother that support lactation and suppress cyclic ovarian function (this acts to decrease the chance of subsequent pregnancy until lactation is complete). Unfortunately, the loss of ovarian function also produces a series of physiological changes that produce multiple side effects that are similar to those seen during menopause (Cunningham et al. 1997). The uterus shrinks rapidly to near its original size, menstrual periods cease temporarily, and the lining of the vagina thins dramatically. Vaginal secretions are scant, and dry skin is common. Bone mineral loss is rapid and substantial (Drinkwater and Chestnut 1991; Little et al. 1993), averaging about 5 percent over the initial three months, and many women experience emotional instability (occasionally losing control over their emotions), hot flashes, and night sweats due to this temporary loss in ovarian function. Unfortunately, continuing regular exercise during the early postpartum period does not appear to influence the timing of the return of ovarian function in lactating women nor does it decrease their rate of bone mineral loss. It does, however, appear to be helpful in reducing the frequency and severity of episodes of emotional instability, hot flashes, and night sweats until ovarian function returns.

The increases in breast size and breast mobility that occur during pregnancy increase further during lactation. Hence, lactating women should obtain adequate stabilization and support of the breasts during exercise. Lactating women should choose support materials with a high percentage of either cotton or silk in the fabric and with no seams to avoid nipple abrasions.

Additional physiological changes that influence exercise prescription and performance occur at a variable rate over the first year after giving birth. The rate appears to be related to hormonal and lifestyle factors, but the pattern of a gradual return of physiological function toward that characteristic of the nonpregnant state is consistent. Cardiovascular, metabolic, endocrine, and thermal responses revert, but the magnitude of the changes are highly variable between women and, in some, both the thermal and cardiovascular changes persist to a significant degree. Potentially, this should give them a competitive edge because both an improved ability to dissipate heat and a higher stroke volume should improve performance. Indeed, factors like this may account for the improved performances seen in some national class women athletes after having a baby.

Tissues and ligaments that surround and support the uterus, bladder, vagina, and rectum involute and shorten. The same is true for the ligaments that surround and stabilize joints in the pelvis, back, hips, and knees. The connective tissue tension and muscular tone of the abdomen improves, and gradual weight loss ensues. Ultimately, in the areas of weight loss and abdominal tone, it takes most active women between six months and one year to return to their prepregnancy state.

Spontaneous Patterns of Exercise Performance After the Birth

When I first started studying exercising women in the early 1980s, I was amazed to find that most of them resumed some form of exercise routine within two weeks after the birth. I didn't understand where they found the time, and I was also concerned that it wasn't a smart thing to do. I'd been taught that women should avoid all physical stress for two weeks (don't drive a car, carry anything heavier than the baby, climb stairs, and so on), and not resume full daily activities for a minimum of six weeks. Incidentally, this was and still is the recommendation of the American College of Obstetricians and Gynecologists (1994). I guess it was assumed that everything (abdomen, uterus, joints, supporting ligaments, vagina, and so on) that had been stretched by the pregnancy and delivery would not shrink back to normal if you stressed it during this *involutional* phase. I'd also heard that excessive movement of the breasts might cause nipple abrasions and interfere with breast-feeding. So I decided we should look at this in our studies, too.

Many active women resume exercise within two weeks after the birth of their babies.

I began by asking the women a few questions, and the answers were surprising. For example, I asked "What did the doctor say about exercise before you left the hospital?" I always got one of three very different answers:

"He didn't say" (don't ask, don't tell).

"Oh, you know she means well, but she's old fashioned" (party line was ignored).

"He says to wait a few days, and after that anything that doesn't hurt or make me bleed heavily is OK" (apparently a popular point of view that these women agreed with).

So who's right?

Next I asked if they weren't concerned they might damage something by exercising so soon after delivery. Clearly, they thought that was foolish. So then I asked why they decided to start so soon. The most common answer was "It feels good, and it gives me personal time away from the baby!"

Then I watched to see what happened as these women exercised. I saw most of the women at regular intervals, and as far as I could tell nothing bad happened. Indeed, they recovered from the delivery quickly and told me that their doctors said everything was OK at their checkups. The same was true for the few who required a cesarean delivery. Likewise, even though over 95 percent breast-fed, they didn't have any problems with their breasts, and they felt well. Over the first year, they lost all excess fat, returned to their prepregnant weight, and their exercise capacity exceeded its prepregnancy level. Since then, we've continued to examine postpartum exercise in greater detail and have drawn the conclusion that, if it doesn't hurt or cause the woman to bleed heavily, it's OK.

At one point, I began designing experiments to help me decide what was the right thing to do, what was the wrong thing to do, and why. I rapidly recognized that I was going to have to cheat a bit. There was no way I was going to be able to get women who exercised throughout their pregnancies to stop exercising after the birth. It was going to be like studying exercise in pregnancy all over again. I'd have to start by learning from what the women did and did not do. So I arranged to keep track of who exercised and who didn't. I saw what worked, what didn't, and what the problems were. In the remainder of this chapter, I've translated that information into some guidelines that can help in designing an exercise program for the first year after the birth. I've divided that time into two parts—the first six weeks after the birth and thereafter—because the problems encountered and the goals set usually change at about the sixth week.

First Six Weeks After the Birth

This is an intense time for a woman. First, she never thought that she would feel this way about another human being, and she needs to adjust to that. Second, she's recovering from the birth. Third, everything is new, she wants to do the right thing, everybody gives her different advice, she's up half the night, and the rest of life is a blur. If you ask her what she needs, she'll tell you—some personal time away from the baby and everyone else, which will allow her to relax and have time to think about things. This personal time is where exercise comes in, and it should be the focus of the exercise program for this time interval. The goals are clear: frequent exercise sessions that provide spaced personal time and relaxation—nothing more, nothing less. A change is necessary only if the woman does not achieve these goals or a problem develops.

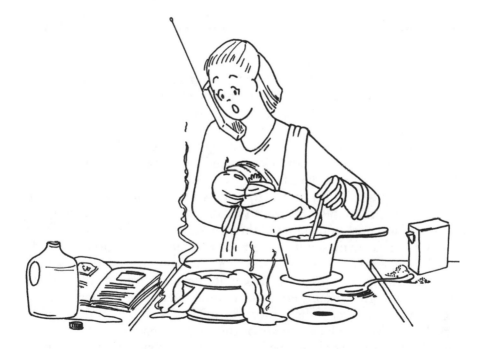

Stressed-out new mother.

Education

Proper exercise education should be quick and to the point. Indeed, after the birth there's so much going on that I try to cover these things during one of the evaluation sessions in late pregnancy. I stress five things.

1. **Time away from the baby and house can keep a woman from feeling overwhelmed.** This time is important because that overwhelmed feeling is the first step toward postpartum depression (estimated to occur in at least one in four women after their first baby), and many women find that exercise is a way to be sure they get that time away.

2. **Paying attention to the baby and herself during this time is important.** If a woman ignores the rest of the world, then there will be plenty of time to take care of both sets of needs. Let the father or other family member worry about the rest for a while. During this hectic time, exercise provides time to relax and think.

3. **Avoiding fatigue.** The easiest way for a new mother to avoid fatigue is by sleeping when the baby sleeps and being awake when the baby's awake. This is simply another version of the rest-activity cycling we've talked about throughout the pregnancy. Why stop now? It also helps to plan one session of awake quiet time for relaxation during the day. Early afternoon is the best.

4. **Drinking a lot of fluids and eating at regular intervals and well.** At this time, lactation plays a major role in most women's lives and, like exercise, it takes extra calories and lots of water. Avoiding dehydration is difficult, and the new mother should increase her intake of carbohydrate as well. A good rule is eight ounces of fluid and a piece of fruit, a salad, or half a sandwich for the mother each time she nurses the baby. The same applies to after exercise.

5. **A woman should think support when she exercises.** Nursing women should double bra (wear two bras) during their exercise sessions to compress and stabilize the breasts on the chest wall. If that doesn't satisfactorily stabilize the breasts, then the addition of a wide Ace bandage crisscrossed over the chest and shoulders with moderate tension usually does the trick. Moderate tension means that it should be tight enough so that there is the definite feeling of support but not tight enough to create discomfort during the workout. If discomfort develops there may be a wrinkle or the support may be too tight. Ideally, the Ace bandage should be between the two bras, but some women with large breasts find it more comfortable applying the Ace bandage over both rather than between the two bras. In the first few weeks after

delivery, exercise causes the lax abdominal wall to bounce and shift as well. Therefore, during this time, I recommend that a woman use either tights or an overgirth or both to support her abdomen.

Focus on establishing a rhythm
and avoiding fatigue and dehydration.

Interactive Component

It's important that a new mother's exercise time occur at a time of day and under circumstances that do not cause her to worry about the baby. She should pick the best time for her (emotionally this usually is midafternoon or early evening). The first few times, she may find it hard to leave the baby, but as she recognizes the benefits, then this becomes easier. Occasionally, timing is a problem (spouse away on business, new community, or the like). Under these circumstances, either an experienced older sitter or a jogging stroller can be wonderful solutions.

Type of Exercise

The rule is start early and increase slowly. Although most active women return to exercise soon after delivery, they don't reach their predelivery performance level for two to three months at least. It usually takes twice that long for them to feel like they did before they got pregnant. For this reason, this phase is usually a difficult time for the serious athlete unless she has lots of help. The message I preach is patience. If she has patience for a couple months, then serious training will make her better than she was before.

After delivery, start frequent sessions of sustained weight-
bearing exercise early and gradually increase exercise volume
(the product of duration and intensity) over time.

In the initial six weeks, the type of exercise doesn't matter too much. I recommend working out at least three times a week; however, five times a week is ideal. Exercising more frequently is OK especially if the woman feels that she needs to get away more, but she shouldn't overdo it at first. The important things are that the exercise is solitary, and it makes the woman sweat a little and feel good. Jogging is ideal. Early morning workouts at the health club are OK, too, but for most, there are too many interruptions from other people during the day and evening.

Swimming and cycling also work well. Some doctors, however, don't want women to swim for several weeks after the birth, because they feel there's an increased risk of infection until healing is complete. Likewise, if the woman required an episiotomy (an incision to make extra room for the birth of the baby), bike riding is usually out of the question for a few months.

Instruction and Safety

The same equipment and environmental rules apply as during pregnancy. The only new safety concern is childcare or appropriate placement of the infant in a jogger, frontpack, or carriage. Most baby joggers are designed like a sling to hold the infant tightly and provide excellent stability for the neck and head; many of the frontpacks do not have this built-in stability and care should be taken to assure that the baby's head, neck, and trunk are stable.

Monitoring

To be sure that things will go well, the woman needs to self-monitor a few things, and the health fitness and health care practitioners should be readily available to deal with questions or concerns. In these first six weeks the important things are as follows:

- The woman should exercise three or more times a week.
- The exercise should feel good and enhance feelings of well-being.
- There should be no exercise-associated pain or heavy bleeding.
- Personal well-being should be self-assessed every two or three days.
- Fluid intake should be high.
- Adequate rest is a must.
- Infant weight gain should be normal.

How much fluid is enough? A good rule of thumb is a woman should drink enough so that she feels she has to urinate every time she feeds the baby and, remember, the urine should be pale to clear.

Fatigue can be a common problem with including an exercise routine after the baby is born. If the new mother is tired all the time, something needs to change. The best way to handle this is to hold a family council to determine what can be done to help. Often, some help from a family member, temporary use of a cleaning service, or ordering dinner out occasionally is all that is needed. But in some instances the exercise program may need revision. Here the important issue is "Does the exercise provide relaxation and enhance well-being?" If the answer is "no" or if there is stiffness, soreness, and fatigue after exercise, then revising the exercise program is necessary. Often the problem is as simple as too high an intensity or forgetting to stretch after each exercise session. Sometimes, it's simply the time of day coupled with overcommitment. If a woman has to set an alarm in order to get up early enough to fit her exercise in, it's the wrong time of day. The same is true if she skips lunch or an afternoon nap! Sometimes a long jog three times a week is too much while a more appropriate program may be half the distance five times a week.

Rarely, the type of exercise needs to be changed. Joint pain that becomes more intense as the session continues and persists afterward is the usual symptom, and the cure is to temporarily reduce the load on the affected joint by changing the activity (e.g., water running, water aerobics, or rowing machine instead of jogging).

Focus on hydration, infant weight gain,
and avoiding pain and fatigue.

I think every woman with a new baby should buy a baby scale. Many worry that their baby might not be getting enough to eat. However, if the baby is not cranky, he or she is getting enough to eat. If the woman wants to be absolutely sure, she can simply weigh the baby every now and then before and after a feeding; then she will know for certain how much milk he or she has consumed and if the rate of weight gain is appropriate (between a quarter and half a pound a week). If the baby is cranky all the time, then the same approach helps to eliminate inadequate milk intake as the cause. An alternate approach, advocated by the La Leche League and the American Academy of Pediatrics, is to count the number of wet and soiled diapers in every 24-hour period (5 to 6 good wet disposable diapers or 6 to 8 cloth coupled with soft stool indicates adequate intake). If these conditions are met, the usual well-baby checks should be sufficient for monitoring weight gain.

Dos and Don'ts

✓ *Do be sure that the amount of exercise is enough but not too much.* It should be enough to improve well-being but not enough to precipitate any of the problems discussed earlier in the chapter.

✓ *Do be sure that exercise feels good.* This rule is valuable throughout the entire reproductive cycle, but especially so during late pregnancy and the initial six weeks after the birth. Physical discomfort and pain are not normal and deserve attention. The adage "no pain, no gain" definitely does not apply at this point in time.

✓ *Do pay attention to the little things.* They are very important during times of change. Stay well hydrated, eat well, and get adequate rest.

✓ *Don't chart performance progress.* This six-week period is the only time that progress in the exercise regimen is not important. A woman should simply adjust her overall exercise volume by how she feels.

✓ *Don't ignore fatigue or pain.*

Contraindications to Exercise

As far as I'm concerned there are three *absolute contraindications* to exercise during the first six weeks after the birth.

1. **Heavy bleeding.** How much is heavy? Copious (a pad every half-hour), bright red bleeding that persists for several hours. If this occurs, the woman should be checked right away to be sure she hasn't accumulated clotted blood in her womb or torn out a stitch. Even if nothing's wrong, she still should wait 48 hours before she tries exercising again.

Heavy bleeding, pain, and infection are the big three contraindications to exercise.

---

2. **Pain.** If it hurts anywhere, stop. Pain means that something is wrong, and it should be checked out before a woman continues.

Usually it means that she needs new shoes, more support, or has over-done it. Correct the problem, then start again at a lower level.

3. **Breast infection or abscess.** If a woman develops a breast infection or abscess, she should consult her physician, stop the exercise, and immobilize the breast until the abscess is drained or the infection resolves. Lots of motion can spread the infection. The same is true if a serious infection occurs in the womb, an incision, or at any other site.

Why should a woman with a new baby take chances with her health? *Relative contraindications* vary from one provider to another, but I think that all would agree on three.

1. **Cesarean birth or traumatic vaginal birth.** There's the question of whether a woman should exercise in the six weeks following a cesarean section delivery or a traumatic vaginal birth (deep tears into the rectal area that required extensive repair). In our experience, some women start back within two weeks; others don't until four weeks or so. The deciding factor is pain. Again, if it hurts, stop, and if it feels good, it's probably OK.

2. **Breast discomfort.** Here the answer is simple—if the woman is engorged, she shouldn't exercise until the engorgement is over. If she's not, more support will probably solve a problem of breast discomfort, but she should have her breasts checked anyway to be sure it's not something more serious.

3. **Heavy urine leakage or pelvic pressure during exercise.** Some leakage and pressure are normal at this time, and the woman should exercise with an empty bladder, wearing a pad. However, if the leakage is heavy or lasts longer than a couple weeks, a health care provider should evaluate it before the woman continues exercise. The same is true for pelvic pressure.

From Six Weeks On

By six weeks after the birth, most women who exercise are beginning to have everything under control. The baby's sleeping most of the night; they're back to work and have developed a new schedule that works. Breast-feeding is now a routine, and the baby is growing and lots of fun. Time is still tight, but life is manageable, especially if she shares her exercise time with the baby (see figures 11.1 and 11.2). If running is part of her training program, purchasing one of the many types of jogging strollers can solve problems and make time she otherwise would not have. As her free time increases (usually about three to four months

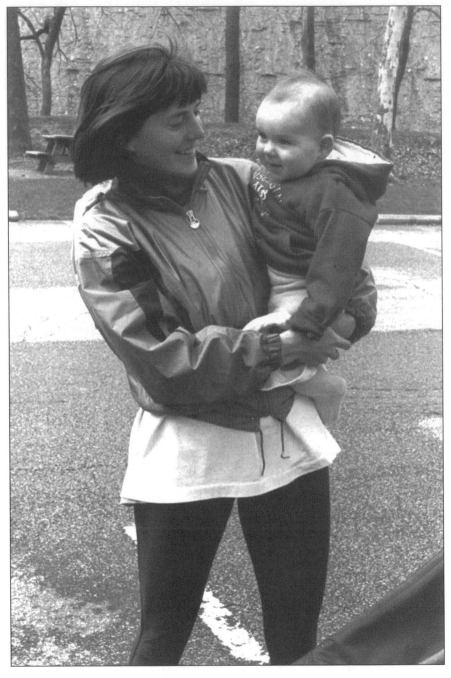

Figure 11.1 Time together.

after the birth), she begins to take stock of where she wants to be six months down the road.

That means it's time to set exercise goals again! At this time, there are three goals that are shared by most active women:

- A return to prepregnancy weight
- A rapid improvement in abdominal tone
- An improved body image

Many women also want to improve their endurance and performance, and a few want to get back in tip-top competitive shape. A woman can achieve either goal in time with a combination of hard work and discipline. The major problem is women want results, but many don't have the time.

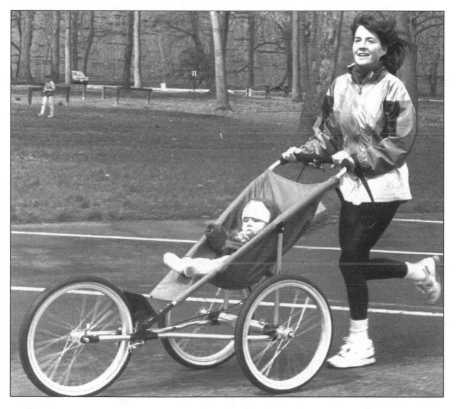

Figure 11.2   Exercise for two.

Exercise Prescription

The key to success is a plan that develops the discipline to find the time for the hard work. If the principles discussed in chapter 8 are applied, this can be achieved, and the rest will be easy. The first step for both the woman and her health fitness instructor is to remember that the exercise regimen must fit into the new lifestyle, then develop an appropriate plan.

Education

The educational component should focus on the value of a balanced, realistic approach (all three components with gradual progression over time) and the dangers of pushing too hard too fast when there is too little time available (overtraining syndrome). The basic message should be—match activity levels and goals with the time available.

Type of Exercise

The health fitness instructor and the woman should work together to tailor the types of exercise to her individual goals, with continued emphasis on a balanced approach that produces easily recognized results. For the best results, the program should include a strength and flexibility component, an endurance component, and usually a skill component. During this phase, there is no reason to restrict specific types of activity, but, as free time is sparse and valuable, focus on activities that do the job as well as being fun and relaxing. Assess progress in the usual way at specified intervals determined by the seriousness of and the timetable for the regimen. The little things are still important and should be monitored, but the acute responses to exercise are no longer a focal point because they're much less important now than they were during the pregnancy.

Monitoring

At this stage, the monitoring should focus on assessing progress in performance. But physical and emotional well-being are always important, and rest-activity cycling should continue as well. The only additional concern is milk production, and the best index of this is the growth and development of the baby. Infant growth charts are helpful but remember that breast-fed babies gain weight a bit more slowly. So as long as the baby is exclusively breast-fed, be sure to use a weight chart that is specific for a breast-fed baby. If the woman doesn't have one in her baby book, then a few questions at each of the well-baby checkups should clarify the issue. Milk production is adequate as long as the baby's growth curves demonstrate normal interval growth. In any case, as long as the mother takes the time to nurse the baby when it is hungry until it is full, milk production and growth should take care of themselves.

Focus monitoring on performance, well-being, and the growth and development of the baby.

In terms of the mother, the most difficult issues involve hydration and rest-activity cycles. The woman needs to be sure there is balance in these two areas. If there isn't enough time for restful, leisurely time with the baby, then mom needs to cut back something else, possibly the exercise program. Monitor hydration status in the usual way. It's extremely important, especially when a rigorous exercise regimen and breast-feeding are combined. Monitor nutritional status by evaluating the rate of weight and fat loss. It should be gradual; usually intake is inadequate if there is a return to prepregnancy weight and fat content in less than six months. Use weekly self-assessment of discomfort, pain, performance, motivation, and fatigue to detect early evidence of over- or undertraining and adjust the training schedule accordingly.

The other important lifestyle decision that needs to be made is how long to continue breast-feeding. In my experience there is no right answer. Once maternity leave is over, continuing to breast-feed around the clock becomes difficult. The usual solution (see figure 11.3) for the motivated woman is to pump during the day whenever she gets a spare minute and breast-feed before and after work. As you can see, even in a hospital, the problem for the career-oriented woman is finding a free breast pump and a little privacy when you have a spare minute. It's hard to relax and let the milk flow when the phone is ringing and your beeper is going off, but it's the only solution for many women. Some reduce the problem by purchasing their own pump, and I am told that a reliable double pump (which speeds pumping time) can be purchased through local chapters of the La Leche League (listed in all phone books). Finally, some women find that they can gradually adjust their milk production so that they can nurse effectively while at home without pumping during the day. This avoids difficulty during the workday yet provides benefit and satisfaction to both the women and their infants.

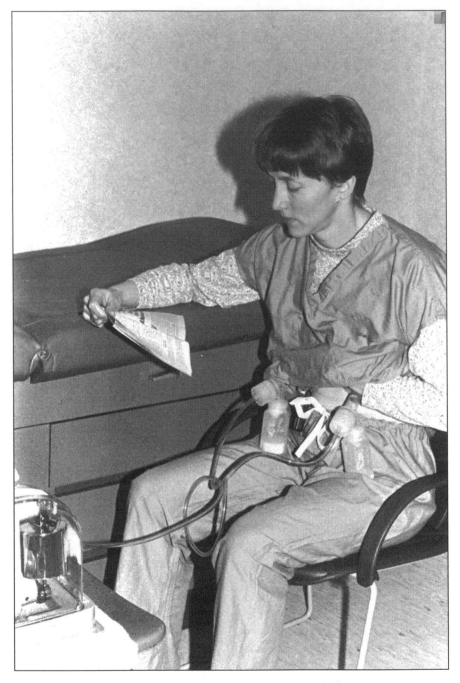

Figure 11.3   Breast pump to the rescue.

The growth rate of the babies of regularly exercising women should be monitored as an exercise variable as long as breast milk is supplying more than 50 percent of the infant's calories. For the remainder of the first year every two to three months is an appropriate interval for the offspring of all three groups of women. Weight, length, and head circumference are the important parameters to measure.

Keep and periodically review a detailed exercise log to ensure that the schedule set out is doing the trick. Look for changes in the relationship between the workload, pulse rate, and the rating of perceived exertion, speed during high mileage workouts, strength, and sport-specific skill. All should improve over time. I recommend also measuring maximal oxygen consumption in the serious athlete at three-month intervals to be sure capacity as well as performance is improving.

Dos and Don'ts

During this phase of the reproductive process the dos and don'ts are no different from those for any nonpregnant woman. The only exception:

✓ *Do monitor the growth of the baby as long as regular exercise and breast-feeding are combined.*

Contraindications to Exercise

There are no special contraindications at this time. We have looked in detail to determine if there are any, and to date we haven't found a single one. However, remember that the standard four (injury, illness, localized pain, and heavy vaginal bleeding) still apply. In that respect, it has been interesting to see if any of these four occur more frequently after having a baby. Theoretically, you can make a good argument that they should, but the fact is, in the populace we have studied, that is simply not the case.

Summary

The main goal of exercise in the initial six weeks after the birth is for the woman to obtain personal time and redevelop a sense of control over her life. To safely accomplish this, she should follow six guidelines. First, begin slowly and increase gradually. Second, avoid excessive fatigue and dehydration. Third, support and compress the abdomen and breasts. Fourth, if it hurts, stop and evaluate. Fifth, if it feels good, it probably is.

Sixth, bright red vaginal bleeding that is heavier than a normal menstrual period should not occur.

The goal of the exercise regimen in the remainder of the first year after birth is to improve various aspects of the individual's physical status. This is best achieved by developing a program that fits her new lifestyle and incorporates components to develop strength and flexibility as well as endurance and sport-specific skills. There are no restrictions other than time on the type and amount of exercise. Monitoring should focus primarily on improvement in performance and progress toward specific goals. Take the usual precautions to avoid overtraining and ensure maternal well-being and adequate growth of the infant throughout.

Epilogue

Well, that's what we now know and have found in research about exercise during conception, pregnancy, lactation, and recovery. I hope you find it helpful, and if your experience turns out to be different from the women I've studied, I'd appreciate it if you would let me know. I can be reached via mail at

> Dr. J.F. Clapp
> c/o MetroHealth Medical Center
> 2500 MetroHealth Drive
> Cleveland, OH 44106

Or via e-mail at **jfclapp@metrohealth.org**.

We're a lot further along now with research on exercise during pregnancy than we were five years ago, and I'm sure that our knowledge will grow exponentially over the next few years. As this knowledge changes, I'll work to update the book. When I look back and recognize how much my ideas and recommendations have changed over the last 10 years, I believe they will continue to change in the future as well.

Because all our current information indicates that exercise during the various phases of reproduction is good, we plan to see if it can't prevent problems from occurring in so-called high-risk pregnancies. My laboratory is focusing on two areas. First, we are trying to determine if regular exercise can prevent premature labor and poor fetal growth in women at the two extremes of reproductive life (for women younger than 16 and older than 35 years of age). Second, we wish to determine if diet and exercise can be used to prevent or treat gestational diabetes. Exercise does help prevent a variety of health problems at other times in life, so why not during pregnancy and lactation? It may turn out that the two most important things a woman can do to ensure a healthy pregnancy with a good outcome are to stop smoking and start exercising before getting pregnant. Only time and more studies will tell.

Appendix

For further information on exercise, pregnancy, and lactation, contact these national organizations.

American College of Obstetricians and
    Gynecologists (ACOG)
600 Maryland Avenue, SW
Suite 300 East
Washington, DC 20024
202-638-5577

American College of Sports Medicine
    (ACSM)
P.O. Box 1440
Indianapolis, IN 46206-1440
317-637-9200

YWCA of the USA
726 Broadway, 5th Floor
New York, NY 10003
212-614-2700

YMCA of the USA
101 North Wacker Drive
Chicago, IL 60606
800-822-9622

La Leche League International
1400 North Meacham Road
Schaumburg, IL 60173
847-519-7730

Melpomene Institute
1010 University Ave.
St. Paul, MN 55104
612-642-1951

Motherwell
1106 Stratford Drive
Carlisle, PA 17013
1-800-MOMWELL

Women's Sport Foundation (WSF)
Eisenhower Park
East Meadow, NY 11554
800-227-3988

Many health clubs, HMOs, and hospitals employ certified fitness instructors to instruct and monitor women's exercise programs during pregnancy and lactation. Additional local resources include women's clubs and sport organizations.

References

Abramson, D., S.M. Robert, and P.D. Wilson. 1934. Relaxation of the pelvic joints in pregnancy. *Surgery Gynecology and Obstetrics* 58: 595-613.

American College of Obstetricians and Gynecologists. 1985. Exercise during pregnancy and the postpartum period. *Technical Bulletin 58*. Washington, DC: ACOG Press.

———. 1994. Exercise during pregnancy and the postpartum period. *Technical Bulletin 189*. Washington, DC: ACOG Press.

American College of Sports Medicine. 1994. *Guidelines for exercise testing and prescription*. Philadelphia: Lea & Febiger.

Artal, R. 1996. Exercise: An alternative therapy for gestational diabetes. *The Physician and Sports Medicine* 24(3): 54-65.

Artal, R., and R.J. Buckenmeyer. 1995. Exercise during pregnancy and postpartum. *Contemporary Obstetrics and Gynecology* 40(5): 62-90.

Artal, R., V. Fortunato, A. Welton, N. Constantino, N. Khodiguian, L. Villalobos, and R. Wiswell. 1995. A comparison of cardiopulmonary adaptations to exercise in pregnancy at sea level and altitude. *American Journal of Obstetrics and Gynecology* 172: 1170-1178.

Artal, R., S. Rutherford, T. Romen, R.K. Kammula, F.J. Dorey, and R.A. Wiswell. 1986. Fetal heart rate responses to maternal exercise. *American Journal of Obstetrics and Gynecology* 155: 729-733.

Artal, R., and R.A. Wiswell. 1986. *Exercise in pregnancy*. Baltimore: Williams & Wilkins.

Ayers, J.W.T., Y. Komesu, T. Romani, and R. Ansbacher. 1985. Anthropomorphic, hormonal and psychologic correlates of semen quality in endurance-trained male athletes. *Fertility and Sterility* 43: 917-921.

Beckmann, C.R.B., and C.A. Beckmann. 1990. Effect of a structured antepartum exercise program on pregnancy and labor outcome in primiparas. *Journal of Reproductive Medicine* 35: 704-709.

Berg, G., M. Hammer, J. Moller-Neison, U. Linden, and J. Thorblad. 1988. Low back pain during pregnancy. *Obstetrics and Gynecology* 71: 71-74.

Berkowitz, G.S., J.L. Kelsey, T.R. Holford, and R.L. Berkowitz. 1983. Physical activity and the risk of spontaneous premature delivery. *Journal of Reproductive Medicine* 28: 581-588.

Borg, G.A.V. 1998. *Borg's perceived exertion and pain scales*. Champaign, IL: Human Kinetics.

Bullen, B.A., G.S. Skrinar, I.Z. Beitins, G. Von Mering, B.A. Turnbull, and J.W. MacArthur. 1985. Induction of menstrual disorders by strenuous exercise in untrained women. *New England Journal of Medicine* 312: 1349-1353.

Burt, C. 1949. Peripheral skin temperature in normal pregnancy. *Lancet* 2: 787-790.

Butte, N.F., C. Garza, E. O'Brien-Smith, and B.L. Nichols. 1984. Human milk intake and growth in exclusively breast-fed infants. *Pediatrics* 104: 187-195.

Calganeri, M., H.A. Bird, and V. Wright. 1982. Changes in joint laxity occurring during pregnancy. *Annals of Rheumatic Disease* 41: 126-128.

Capeless, E.L., and J.F. Clapp. 1989. Cardiovascular changes in early phase of pregnancy. *American Journal of Obstetrics and Gynecology* 161: 1449-1453.

Carpenter, M.W., S.P. Sady, B. Hoegsberg, M.A. Sady, B. Haydon, E.M. Cullinane, D.R. Coustan, and P.D. Thompson. 1988. Fetal heart rate response to maternal exertion. *Journal of the American Medical Association* 259: 3000-3009.

Carpenter, M.W., S.P. Sady, M.A. Sady, B. Haydon, D.R. Coustan, and P.D. Thompson. 1990. Effect of maternal weight gain during pregnancy on exercise performance. *Journal of Applied Physiology* 68: 1173-1176.

Clapp, J.F. 1980. Acute exercise stress in the pregnant ewe. *American Journal of Obstetrics and Gynecology* 136: 489-494.

————. 1985a. Fetal heart rate response to running in midpregnancy and late pregnancy. *American Journal of Obstetrics and Gynecology* 153: 251-252.

————. 1985b. Maternal heart rate in pregnancy. *American Journal of Obstetrics and Gynecology* 152: 659-660.

————. 1987. The effects of exercise on uterine blood flow. In *Uterine blood flow*, ed. C.R. Rosenfeld, 300-310. Ithaca: Perinatology Press.

————. 1989a. The effects of maternal exercise on early pregnancy outcome. *American Journal of Obstetrics and Gynecology* 161: 1453-1457.

————. 1989b. Oxygen consumption during treadmill exercise before, during, and after pregnancy. *American Journal of Obstetrics and Gynecology* 161: 1458-1464.

————. 1991. The changing thermal response to endurance exercise during pregnancy. *American Journal of Obstetrics and Gynecology* 165: 1684-1689.

————. 1994a. A clinical approach to exercise during pregnancy. *Clinics in Sports Medicine* 13: 443-457.

————. 1994b. Physiological adaptation to intrauterine growth retardation. In *Early fetal growth and development*, ed. R.N.T. Ward, S.K. Smith, and D. Donnai, 371-382. London: RCOG Press.

————. 1996a. Exercise during pregnancy. In *Perspectives in exercise science and sports medicine*. Vol. 9, *Exercise and the female—A lifespan approach*, ed. O. Bar-Or, D. Lamb, and P. Clarkson, 413-451. Carmel, IN: Cooper.

————. 1996b. The morphometric and neurodevelopmental outcome at five years of age of the offspring of women who continued to exercise throughout pregnancy. *Journal of Pediatrics* 129: 856-863.

————. 1996c. Pregnancy outcome: Physical activities inside versus outside the workplace. *American Journal of Perinatology* 20: 70-76.

————. 1997. Diet, exercise, and feto-placental growth. *Arcives Gynecologie and Obstetrics* 261: 101-107.

Clapp, J.F., and E.L. Capeless. 1990. Neonatal morphometrics following endurance exercise during pregnancy. *American Journal of Obstetrics and Gynecology* 163: 1805-1811.

————. 1991a. The changing glycemic response to exercise during pregnancy. *American Journal of Obstetrics and Gynecology* 165: 1678-1683.

————. 1991b. The VO_2max of recreational athletes before and after pregnancy. *Medicine and Science in Sports and Exercise* 23: 1128-1133.

Clapp, J.F., E.L. Capeless, K.H. Rizk, and S. Appleby-Wineberg. 1995. The vascular remodelling of pregnancy persists 1 year postpartum. *Journal of the Society for Gynecologic Investigation* 2: 292.

Clapp, J.F., and S. Dickstein. 1984. Endurance exercise and pregnancy outcome. *Medicine and Science in Sports and Exercise* 16: 556-562.

Clapp, J.F., and K.D. Little. 1995. The effect of endurance exercise on pregnancy weight gain and subcutaneous fat deposition. *Medicine and Science in Sports and Exercise* 27: 170-177.

Clapp, J.F., K.D. Little, S.K. Appleby-Wineberg, and J.A. Widness. 1995. The effect of regular maternal exercise on erythropoietin in cord blood and amniotic fluid. *American Journal of Obstetrics and Gynecology* 172: 1445-1450.

Clapp, J.F., K.D. Little, and E.L. Capeless. 1993. Fetal heart rate response to various intensities of recreational exercise during mid and late pregnancy. *American Journal of Obstetrics and Gynecology* 168: 198-206.

Clapp, J.F., and K.H. Rizk. 1992. Effect of recreational exercise on mid-trimester placental growth. *American Journal of Obstetrics and Gynecology* 167: 1518-1521.

Clapp, J.F., B.L. Seaward, R.H. Sleamaker, and J. Hiser. 1988. Maternal physiologic adaptations to early human pregnancy. *American Journal of Obstetrics and Gynecology* 159: 1456-1460.

Clapp, J.F., S.J. Simonian, R.A. Harcar-Sevcik, B. Lopez, and S. Appleby-Wineberg. 1995. Morphometric and neurodevelopmental outcome after exercise during pregnancy. *Medicine and Science in Sports and Exercise* 27: S74.

Clapp, J.F., J. Tomaselli, S. Appleby-Wineberg, S.E. Ridzon, B. Lopez, C. Cowap, and K.D. Little. 1996. Training volume during pregnancy—Effect on fetal heart rate response, maternal weight gain, and fat deposition. *Medicine and Science in Sports and Exercise* 28: S60.

Clapp, J.F. , J. Tomaselli, S. Rizdon, M. Kortan, B. Lopez, and K.D. Little. 1997. Pregnancy training volume—Effect on placental growth and size at birth. *Medicine and Science in Sports and Exercise* 29: S4.

Clapp, J.F., M. Wesley, and R.H. Sleamaker. 1987. Thermoregulatory and metabolic responses to jogging prior to and during pregnancy. *Medicine and Science in Sports and Exercise* 19: 124-130.

Coggan, A.R., W.M. Kohrt, R.J. Sina, D.M. Bier, and J.O. Holloszy. 1990. Endurance training decreases glucose turnover and oxidation during moderate intensity exercise in men. *Journal of Applied Physiology* 68: 990-996.

Cohen, G.C., J.C. Prior, Y. Vigna, and S.M. Pride. 1989. Intense exercise during the first two trimesters of unapparent pregnancy. *The Physician and Sportsmedicine* 17: 87-94.

Collings, C.A., L.B. Curet, and J.P. Mullen. 1983. Maternal and fetal responses to a maternal aerobic exercise program. *American Journal of Obstetrics and Gynecology* 146: 702-707.

Cunningham, F.G., P.C. MacDonald, N.F. Gant, L.C. Gilstrap, G.D.V. Hankins, and S.L. Clark. Eds. 1997. *Williams Obstetrics* (20th ed.) Stamford, CT: Appelton and Lange, 533-546.

Dale, E., K.M. Mullinax, and D.H. Bryan. 1982. Exercise during pregnancy: Effects on the fetus. *Canadian Journal of Applied Sports Science* 7: 98-102.

Dempsey, J.A., and R. Fregosi. 1985. Adaptability of the pulmonary system to changing metabolic requirements. *American Journal of Cardiology* 55: 59D-67D.

DeSwiet, M. 1991. The respiratory system. In *Clinical physiology in obstetrics*, ed. F. Hytten and G. Chamberlain, 83-100. London: Blackwell Scientific.

Dewey, K.G., M.J. Heinig, L.A. Nommsen, J.M. Peerson, and B. Lonnerdal. 1991. Adequacy of energy intake among breast-fed infants in the DARLING study: Relationships to growth velocity, morbidity, and activity levels. *Journal of Pediatrics* 119: 538-547.

———. 1992. Growth of breast-fed and formula fed infants from 0 to 18 months: The DARLING study. *Pediatrics* 89: 1035-1041.

———. 1993. Breast-fed infants are leaner than formula-fed infants at 1 y of age: The DARLING study. *American Journal of Clinical Nutrition* 57: 140-145.

Dewey, K.G., and C.A. Lovelady. 1993. Exercise and breast-feeding: A different experience. *Pediatrics* 91: 514-515.

Dewey, K.G., C.A. Lovelady, L.A. Nommsen-Rivers, M.A. McCrory, and B. Lonnerdal. 1994. A randomized study of the effects of aerobic exercise by lactating women on breast-milk volume and composition. *New England Journal of Medicine* 330: 449-453.

Dewey, K.G., and M.A. McCrory. 1994. Effects of dieting and physical activity on pregnancy and lactation. *American Journal of Clinical Nutrition* 59: 446S-453S.

Dewey, K.G., J.M. Peerson, K.H. Brown, N.F. Krebs, K.F. Michaelsen, L.A. Peerson, L. Salmenpera, R.G. Whitehead, and D.L. Yeung. 1995. Growth of breast-fed infants deviates from current reference data: A pooled analysis of US, Canadian, and European data sets. *Pediatrics* 96: 495-503.

Dewey, K.J., R.J. Cohen, L.L. Rivera, J. Canahuati, and K.H. Brown. 1996. Do exclusively fed breast-fed infants require extra protein? *Pediatric Research* 39: 303-307.

Drinkwater, B.L., and C.H. Chestnut III. 1991. Bone density changes during pregnancy and lactation in active women. *Bone Mineral* 14: 153-160.

Drinkwater, B.L., K. Milson, C.H. Chestnut III, W.J. Bremner, S. Shainholtz, and M.B. Southworth. 1984. Bone mineral content of amenorrheic and eumenorrheic runners. *New England Journal of Medicine* 311: 277-281.Duvekot, J.J., E.C. Cheriex, F.A. Pieters, P.P. Menheere, and L.H. Peeters. 1993. Early pregnancy changes in hemodynamics and volume homeostasis are consecutive adjustments triggered by a primary fall in vascular tone. *American Journal of Obstetrics and Gynecology* 169: 1382-1392.

Eichner, E.R. 1992. Exercise and testicular function. *Sports Science Exchange* 5(38).

Ellis, M.I., B.B. Seedhom, and V. Wright. 1985. Forces in women 36 weeks pregnant and four weeks after delivery. *Engineering Medicine* 14: 95-99.

Erdelyi, G.J. 1962. Gynecological survey of female athletes. *Journal of Sports Medicine and Physical Fitness* 2: 174-179.

Falk, L.J. 1983. Intermediate sojourners in high altitude: Selection and clinical observations. *Adjustment to High Altitude*. NIH Publication, No. 83-2496, 13-18. Washington, DC: U.S. Department of Health and Human Services.

Frisch, R.E., and J.W. MacArthur. 1974. Menstrual cycles: Fatness as a determinant of minimum weight for height necessary for their maintenance or onset. *Science* 185: 949-951.

Gollnick, P.D. 1985. Metabolism of substrates: Energy substrate metabolism during exercise and as modified by training. *Federation Proceedings* 44: 353-357.

Gollnick, P.D., B.F. Timson, R.L. Moore, and M. Riedy. 1981. Muscular enlargement and number of fibers in skeletal muscles of rat. *Journal of Applied Physiology* 50: 936-943.

Grimby, G. 1965. Renal clearances during prolonged supine exercise at different exercise loads. *Journal of Applied Physiology* 20: 1294-1298.

Hagberg, J.M., J.E. Yerg II, and D.R. Seals. 1988. Pulmonary function in younger and older athletes and untrained men. *Journal of Applied Physiology* 65: 101-105.

Hall, D.C., and D.A. Kaufmann. 1987. Effects of aerobic strength and conditioning on pregnancy outcomes. *American Journal of Obstetrics and Gynecology* 157: 1199-1203.

Hart, M.V., M.J. Morton, J.D. Hosenpud, and J. Metcalfe. 1986. Aortic function during normal human pregnancy. *American Journal of Obstetrics and Gynecology* 154: 887-891.

Hatch, C.M., X.O. Shu, D.E. McLean, B. Levin, M. Begg, L. Reuss, and M. Susser. 1993. Maternal exercise during pregnancy, physical fitness, and fetal growth. *American Journal of Epidemiology* 137: 1105-1114.

Hatoum, N., J.F. Clapp, M.R. Neuman, N. Dajani, S.B. Amini. 1997. Effects of maternal exercise on fetal activity in late gestation. *The Journal of Maternal-Fetal Medicine* 6: 134-139.

Heaney, R.P., and T.G. Skillman. 1971. Calcium metabolism in normal human pregnancy. *Journal of Clinical Endocrinology and Metabolism* 33: 661-676.

Henriksson, J. 1977. Training induced adaptation of skeletal muscle and metabolism during submaximal exercise. *Journal of Physiology* 270: 661-675.

Higdon, H. 1981. Running through pregnancy. *The Runner* 4(3): 46-51.

Huel, G., S. Gueguen, R.C. Bouyer, E. Papiernik, N. Mamelle, B. Laumon, F. Munoz, and D. Collin. 1989. Effective prevention of preterm birth: The French experience measured at Haguenau. *Birth Defects: Original Article Series* 25: 1-234.

Hunscher, H.A., and W.T. Tompkins. 1970. The influence of maternal nutrition on the immediate and long-term outcome of pregnancy. *Clinics in Obstetrics and Gynecology* 13: 130-144.

Hytten, F.E. 1991. The alimentary system. In *Clinical physiology in obstetrics*, ed. F.E. Hytten and G. Chamberlain, 137-149. London: Blackwell Scientific.

Jackson, M.A., P. Gott, S.J. Lye, J.W. Knox Ritchie, and J.F. Clapp. 1995. The effect of maternal aerobic exercise on human placental development: Placental volumetric composition and surface areas. *Placenta* 16: 179-191.

Jarrett, J.C., and W.N. Spellacy. 1984. Jogging during pregnancy: An improved outcome? *Obstetrics and Gynecology* 61: 705-709.

Karzel, R.P., and M.C. Friedman. 1991. Orthopedic injuries in pregnancy. In *Exercise in Pregnancy*, ed. R.A. Artal, R.A. Wiswell, and B.L. Drinkwater, 123-132. Baltimore: Williams & Wilkins.

Katz, M., and M.M. Sokal. 1980. Skin perfusion in pregnancy. *American Journal of Obstetrics and Gynecology* 137: 30-33.

King, J.C., N.F. Butte, M.N. Bronstein, L.E. Kopp, and S.A. Lindquist. 1994. Energy metabolism during pregnancy: Influence of maternal energy status. *American Journal of Clinical Nutrition* 59 (Supplement): 439-445.

Klebanoff, M.A., P.H. Shiono, and J.C. Carey. 1990. The effect of physical activity during pregnancy on preterm delivery and birth weight. *American Journal of Obstetrics and Gynecology* 163: 1450-1456.

Kulpa, P.J., B.M. White, and R. Visscher. 1987. Aerobic exercise in pregnancy. *American Journal of Obstetrics and Gynecology* 156: 1395-1403.

Lamb, R., M. Anderson, and J. Walters. 1979. The effects of forced exercise on two-year-old Holstein heifers. *Journal of Dairy Science* 62: 1791-1797.

Little, K.D., J.F. Clapp, and P.D. Gott. 1993. Bone density changes during pregnancy and lactation in exercising women. *Medicine and Science in Sports and Exercise* 25(Supplement 1): 154.

Little, K.D., J.F. Clapp, and S.E. Ridzon. 1994. Effect of exercise on post partum weight and subcutaneous fat loss. *Medicine and Science in Sports and Exercise* 26(Supplement): 15.

————. 1995. Effect of exercise on body composition changes from pre-pregnancy to three months post partum. *Medicine and Science in Sports and Exercise* 27(Supplement): 170.

Lokey, E.A., Z.V. Tran, C.L. Wells, B.C. Myers, and A.C. Tran. 1991. Effect of physical exercise on pregnancy outcomes: A meta-analytic review. *Medicine and Science in Sports and Exercise* 23: 1234-1239.

Lotgering, F.K., R.D. Gilbert, and L.D. Longo. 1983a. Exercise responses in pregnant sheep: Blood gases, temperatures and fetal cardiovascular system. *Journal of Applied Physiology* 55: 842-850.

————. 1983b. Exercise responses in pregnant sheep: Oxygen consumption, uterine blood flow and blood volume. *Journal of Applied Physiology* 55: 834-841.

————. 1985. Maternal and fetal responses to exercise during pregnancy. *Physiological Reviews* 65: 1-36.

Lotgering, F.K., M.B. Van Dorn, P.C. Struijk, J. Pool, and H.C.S. Wallenburg. 1991. Maximal aerobic exercise in pregnant women: Heart rate, O_2 consumption, CO_2 production and ventilation. *Journal of Applied Physiology* 70: 1016-1023.

Loucks, A.B. 1996. The reproductive system. In *Perspectives in exercise science and sports medicine.* Vol. 9, *Exercise and the female—A lifespan approach,* ed. O. Bar-Or, D. Lamb, and P. Clarkson, 41-72. Carmel, IN: Cooper.

Loucks, A.B., G.A. Laughlin, J.F. Mortola, L. Girton, and S.S.C. Yen. 1992. Hypothalamic-pituitary-thyroidal function in eumenorrheic and amenorrheic athletes. *Journal of Clinical Endocrinology and Metabolism* 75: 514-518.

Loucks, A.B., J.F. Mortola, L. Girton, and S.S.C. Yen. 1989. Alterations in the hypothalamic-pituitary-ovarian and the hypothalamic-pituitary-adrenal axes in athletic women. *Journal of Clinical Endocrinology and Metabolism* 68: 402-411.

Lovelady, C.A., B. Lonnerdal, and K.D. Dewey. 1990. Lactation performance of exercising women. *American Journal of Clinical Nutrition* 52: 103-109.

Luke, B., M. Mamelle, L. Keith, F. Munoz, J. Minogue, E. Papiernik, and T.R.B. Johnson. 1995. The association between occupational factors and preterm birth: A United States study. *American Journal of Obstetrics and Gynecology* 173: 849-862.

Mackinnon, L.T. 1992. *Exercise and immunology.* Champaign, IL: Human Kinetics.

Mamelle, M., B. Laumon, and P. Lazar. 1984. Prematurity and occupational activity during pregnancy. *American Journal of Epidemiology* 119: 309-322.

Marshall, L.A. 1994. Clinical evaluation of amenorrhea in active and athletic women. *Clinics in Sports Medicine* 13(2): 371-387.

McGinnis, J.M. 1992. The public health burden of a sedentary lifestyle. *Medicine and Science in Sports and Exercise* 24: S196-S200.

Melpomene Institute and USMS Sports Medicine Research Committee. 1989. Exercise and pregnancy. *Swim Magazine* May-June: 12-15.

Naeye, R.L., and E.C. Peters. 1982. Work during pregnancy: Effects on the fetus. *Pediatrics* 69: 724-727.

Nisell, H., P. Hjemdahl, and B. Linde. 1985. Cardiovascular responses to circulating catecholamines in normal pregnancy and in pregnancy-induced hypertension. *Clinical Physiology* 5: 479-493.

Oshida, Y., K. Yamanouchi, S. Hayamizu, and Y. Sato. 1989. Long-term mild jogging increases insulin action despite no influence on body mass index or VO_2max. *Journal of Applied Physiology* 66: 2206-2210.

Östgaard, H.C., G. Zetherström, E. Roos-Hansson, and B. Svanberg. 1994. Reduction of back and posterior pelvic pain in pregnancy. *Spine* 19: 894-900.

Pernoll, M.L., J. Metcalfe, T.L. Schlenker, J.E. Welch, and J.A. Matsumoto. 1975. Oxygen consumption at rest and during exercise in pregnancy. *Respiratory Physiology* 25: 285-294.

Pivarnik, J.M., N.A. Ayers, M.B. Mauer, D.B. Cotton, B. Kirshon, and G.A. Dildy. 1993. Effects of maternal aerobic fitness on cardiorespiratory responses to exercise. *Medicine and Science in Sports and Exercise* 25: 993-998.

Pivarnik, J.M., W. Lee, T. Spillman, S.L. Clark, D.B. Cotton, and J.F. Miller. 1992. Maternal respiration and blood gasses during aerobic exercise performed at moderate altitude. *Medicine and Science in Sports and Exercise* 24: 868-872.

Pivarnik, J.M., M.B. Mauer, N.A. Ayres, B. Kirshon, G.A. Dildy, and D.B. Cotton. 1994. Effect of chronic exercise on blood volume expansion and hematologic indices during pregnancy. *Obstetrics and Gynecology* 83: 265-269.

Quinn, T.J., and G.B. Carey. 1997. Is breast milk composition in lactating women altered by exercise intensity or diet? *Medicine and Science in Sports and Exercise* 29: S4.

Rabkin, C.S., H.R. Anderson, J.M. Bland, O.G. Brooke, G. Chamberlain, and J.L. Peacock. 1990. Maternal activity and birth weight: A prospective population-based study. *American Journal of Epidemiology* 131: 522-531.

Reuschlien, P.L., W.G. Reddan, J.F. Burpee, J.B.L. Gee, and J. Rankin. 1968. The effect of physical training on the pulmonary diffusing capacity during submaximal work. *Journal of Applied Physiology* 24: 152-158.

Roberts, M.F., C.B. Wenger, J.A.J. Stolwijk, and E.R. Nadel. 1977. Skin blood flow and sweating changes following exercise training and heat acclimation. *Journal of Applied Physiology* 43: 133-137.

Roberts, S.B., T.J. Cole, and W.A. Coward. 1985. Lactational performance in relation to energy intake in the baboon. *American Journal of Clinical Nutrition* 41: 1270-1276.

Robson, S.C., S. Hunter, R.J. Boys, and W. Dunlop. 1989. Serial study of factors influencing changes in cardiac output during human pregnancy. *American Journal of Physiology* 256: H1060-H1065.

Rowell, L.B. 1974. Human cardiovascular adjustments to exercise and thermal stress. *Physiological Reviews* 54: 75-159.

Ryan, E.A., M.J. O'Sullivan, and J.S. Skyler. 1985. Insulin action during pregnancy: Studies with the euglycemic clamp technique. *Diabetes* 34: 380-389.

Saltin, B., G. Blomqvist, J.H. Mitchell, R.L. Johnson, Jr., K. Wildenthal, and C.B. Chapman. 1968. Response to exercise after bed rest and after training: A longitudinal study of adaptive changes in oxygen transport and body composition. *Circulation* 38 (Supplement 7): 1-78.

Saltin, B., and L. Hermansen. 1966. Esophageal, rectal and muscle temperature during exercise. *Journal of Applied Physiology* 21: 1757-1762.

Saltin, B., and L.B. Rowell. 1980. Functional adaptations to physical activity and inactivity. *Federation Proceedings* 39: 1506-1513.

Sanborn, C.E., B.H. Albrecht, and W.W. Wagner. 1987. Athletic amenorrhea: Lack of association with body fat. *Medicine and Science in Sports and Exercise* 19: 207-212.

Schauberger, C.W., B.L. Rooney, L. Goldsmith, D. Shenton, P.D. Silva, and A. Schaper. 1996. Peripheral joint laxity increases in pregnancy but does not correlate with serum relaxin levels. *American Journal of Obstetrics and Gynecology* 174: 667-671.

Schultz, L.O., A.I. Harper, J.H. Wilmore, and E. Ravussin. 1992. Energy expenditure of elite female runners measured by respiratory chamber and doubly labeled water. *Journal of Applied Physiology* 72: 23-28.

Sherer, D.M., and J.G. Schenker. 1989. Accidental injury during pregnancy. *Obstetrical and Gynecological Survey* 44: 330-338.

Sibley, L., R.O. Ruhling, J. Cameron-Foster, C. Christensen, and T. Bolen. 1981. Swimming and physical fitness during pregnancy. *Journal of Nurse Midwifery* 26: 3-12.

Snellen, J.W. 1969. Body temperature during exercise. *Medicine and Science in Sports and Exercise* 1: 39-44.

South-Paul, J.E., K.R. Rajagopal, and T.F. Tenholder. 1988. The effect of participation in a regular exercise program upon aerobic capacity during pregnancy. *Obstetrics and Gynecology* 71: 175-178.

Sowers, M., M. Crutchfield, M. Jannausch, S. Updike, and G. Corton. 1991. A prospective evaluation of bone mineral change in pregnancy. *Obstetrics and Gynecology* 77: 841-845.

Stephanick, M.L. 1993. Exercise and weight control. *Exercise and Sports Science Reviews* 21: 363-396.

Stephenson, L.A., and M.A. Kolka. 1985. Menstrual cycle phase and time of day alter reference signal controlling arm blood flow and sweating. *American Journal of Physiology* 249: R186-R191.

Strode, M.A., K.G. Dewey, and B. Lonnerdal. 1986. Effects of short-term caloric restriction on lactational performance of well-nourished women. *Acta Paediatrica Scandinavia* 75: 222-229.

Tankersley, C.G., W.C. Nicholas, D.R. Deaver, D. Mitka, and W.L. Kenney. 1992. Estrogen replacement in middle-aged women: Thermoregulatory responses to exercise in the heat. *Journal of Applied Physiology* 73: 1238-1245.

Tipton, C.M., A.C. Vailas, and R.D. Matthes. 1986. Experimental studies on the influences of physical activity on ligaments, tendons, and joints: A brief review. *Acta Medica Scandinavia* (Supplement 711): 157-168.

van Raaij, J.M.A., C.M. Schonk, S.H. Vermaat-Miedema, M.E.M. Peek, and J.G.A.J. Hautvast. 1990. Energy cost of walking at a fixed pace before, during and after pregnancy. *American Journal of Clinical Nutrition* 51: 158-161.

Villarosa, L. 1985. Running and pregnancy: Having it all. *The Runner* 8(7): 25-31.

Wallace, A.M., D.B. Boyer, A. Dan, and K. Holm. 1986. Aerobic exercise, maternal self-esteem, and physical discomforts during pregnancy. *Journal of Nurse Midwifery* 31: 255-262.

Wallace, J.P., G. Inbar, and K. Ernsthausen. 1992. Infant acceptance of postexercise breast milk. *Pediatrics* 89: 1245-1247.

———. 1994. Lactate concentrations in breast milk following maximal exercise and a typical workout. *Journal of Women's Health* 3: 91-96.

Warren, M.P. 1980. The effect of exercise on pubertal progression and reproductive function in girls. *Journal of Clinical Endocrinology and Metabolism* 51: 1150-1157.

Wolfe, L.A., and M.F. Mottola. 1993. Aerobic exercise in pregnancy: An update. *Canadian Journal of Applied Physiology* 18: 119-147.

Wolfe, L.A., R.M.C. Walker, A. Bonen, and M.J. McGrath. 1994. Respiratory adaptations to acute and chronic exercise in pregnancy. *Journal of Applied Physiology* 76: 1928-1936.

Wong, S.C., and D.C. McKenzie. 1987. Cardiorespiratory fitness during pregnancy and its effects on outcome. *International Journal of Sports Medicine* 8: 79-83.

Zaharieva, E. 1972. Olympic participation by women. *Journal of the American Medical Association* 221: 92-95.

Index

Note: Page numbers in *italics* refer to tables

A

abdominal support 88, 92, 200–201, 211
abdominal tone 90, 91, 105, 207
abdominal trauma risk 203
abortion, spontaneous 54–55
aerobic capacity 31, 39, 96–98, 103, 133
aerobics 62, 88, 131, 145, 162
altitudes, exercising in 185, 203
amenorrhea 155, 158
American Academy of Pediatrics 213
American College of Obstetricians and Gynecologists (ACOG)
    address 224
contraindications to exercise 150–151, *151*
guidelines for exercise 6, 136, *137*, 141, 201, 207
American College of Sports Medicine 224
amniotomy 93
amount of exercise
    and ceiling effect 133–134
    and dose-response effect 134
    and duration 132
    and exercise type 131–132
    and frequency 132–133
    and goals 135–136
    and intensity 133
    modifying 198–200, 213
    and overtraining 134–135
    and stages of pregnancy 130–131
    and threshold effect 133–134
Anderson, M. 73–74
animal studies 4–6, 11, 73–74, 76
anovulation 155, 178–179
asthma, exercise-induced 30–31
athletes. *See* beginning exercisers; competitive athletes; Olympic athletes;
    recreational athletes
attitudes
    of competitive athletes 174, 204
    positive 98–102
avoidance response, to exercise 9–10

B

back pain 43
Bayley Test of Infant Development 120
beginning exercisers
    dos and don'ts for 165–167
    education of 158–160, 193

About the Author

James F. Clapp, III, M.D., is an international authority on the effects of exercise during pregnancy. Dr. Clapp is Emeritus Professor of Reproductive Biology at Case Western Reserve University and Research Professor of Obstetrics and Gynecology at the University of Vermont College of Medicine. His ongoing research projects include: follow-up studies of women (and their offspring) who ran, cross-country skied, or performed aerobics throughout their pregnancies 18 to 20 years ago, studies of the effects of additional forms of exercise such as swimming, spinning, and weight training; and studies of the effects of vigorous exercise at high altitude during late pregnancy. Dr. Clapp is a member of The Partnership for an Active Healthy Pregnancy, a group of consumer advocates interested in women's health.

Dr. Clapp completed his medical degree at the University of Vermont College of Medicine. He received research training in pathology at the University of Vermont College of Medicine and training in reproductive physiology at the University of Florida School of Medicine and at Yale University School of Medicine. In the early 1970s Dr. Clapp joined the faculty of the University of Vermont College of Medicine, where he began a series of research projects designed to determine the effects of maternal lifestyle factors on fetal growth and development. In the early 1980s he began a series of comprehensive studies that have examined the effects of maternal exercise on the course and outcome of pregnancy. In 1990 he moved from Vermont to Cleveland, Ohio, where he was the director of obstetrical research at Metro Health Medical Center and a Professor of reproductive biology at Case Western Reserve University School of Medicine.

In his leisure time, Dr. Clapp enjoys running, cross-country skiing, hiking, and spending time with his grandchildren. He and his wife, Nancy, have homes in Byron, California and South Hero, Vermont.

To Order Books

Please send:

_____copies of _____

at $_____ . ____ each.   Total_____

Nebraska residents add 6.5% sales tax   _____

Shipping/Handling
   $4.00 for first book
   $1.00 for each additional book   _____

TOTAL ENCLOSED_____

Name_____

Address_____

City_____State_____Zip_____

☐ Visa   ☐ Mastercard   ☐ American Express

Credit card number_____

Expiration date_____

Order by credit card, personal check, or money order.
Send to:

Addicus Books
P.O. Box 45327
Omaha, NE 68145

Order **TOLL FREE: 800-352-2873**

or online at
www.AddicusBooks.com